Medical Jurisprudence, Insanity, and Toxicology

Medical Jurisprudence, Insanity, and Toxicology

By

HENRY C. CHAPMAN, M.D.

BeardBooks

Washington, D.C.

CONTENTS.

PART I.—MEDICAL JURISPRUDENCE.

CHAPTER I.

CHAPTER II.

CHAPTER III.

CHAPTER IV.

CHAPTER V.

8 Contents.

Contents. 9

PART II.—INSANITY.

PART III.—TOXICOLOGY.

CHAPTER I.

CHAPTER II.

PART I.

MEDICAL JURISPRUDENCE.

PART I.

MEDICAL JURISPRUDENCE.

CHAPTER I.

Importance of the Subject of Medical Jurisprudence—Ordinary and Expert Witnesses—The Coroner's Physician—Relations of the Medical Profession to the Coroner in Cases of Sudden Death, etc.

MEDICAL JURISPRUDENCE, or Forensic Medicine, or Legal Medicine, as the subject is often also called, may be broadly defined as medicine in relation to law. Although a subject of very wide scope and much practical importance, it is, nevertheless, usually neglected by the students of medicine. It is very desirable, however, that every physician should have some knowledge of medical jurisprudence, as he is liable to be called upon at any time during the course of his professional career to give testimony in cases of rape, fœticide, infanticide, death from poison, and from other causes. The physician should know, therefore, what the Commonwealth expects of him and has a right to demand of him in his professional capacity, and he should know his own rights as a medical expert.

Witnesses, however, are of two kinds: One is a witness in the ordinary acceptation of the term who testifies simply to matters of fact of which he has personal knowledge. The other is a witness who likewise testifies to matters of fact, but concerning which he has special professional expert knowledge, such as the ordinary witness cannot, from the nature of the case, be expected to have. A person, for example, happens to be walking in the street. He sees a boy run over by a street car, or a man plunge a dirk into another; or the shot of a pistol is heard and a man is seen to fall. This person is a witness in the ordinary acceptation of the term. That is to say, he is liable by the law of the Commonwealth to be at any time subpœnaed to testify in court to these facts. Such subpœna, when served, the witness must obey. Every citizen may be called upon to testify to matters of fact of which he has personal knowledge. The medical expert witness, however, is of a kind different from the ordinary witness. He is called upon by the prosecution or defense to give an opinion or testimony as to facts of which he has no personal knowledge, but concerning which he is especially qualified to express an opinion on account of his professional training. His knowledge of the particular facts of a case, however, will depend entirely as to whether he sees proper to make himself acquainted with them or not. No law can compel, for example, a physician to examine the contents of a stomach, with the view of determining whether they contain a poison, if he refuses to do so. The physician can excuse himself on the ground that he does not feel competent to make the chemical analysis, or that the necessities of his practice do not give him sufficient time to make such analysis, or that giving testimony in court at the time of the trial may interfere with other professional engagements, etc. The physician may give any such reasons he pleases for refusing to undertake a medico-legal investigation, and no law can compel him to do so.

Ordinarily it would be unwise for a young physician not to avail himself of an opportunity of giving testimony in court, since it undoubtedly leads indirectly to a great deal of practice and professional preferment generally. If the physician does accept this responsibility, it is important that he should know exactly what his duties will be to the Commonwealth under these circumstances, and also what he may expect from the Commonwealth.

Coroner's Physicians.—Usually in every large city there are appointed by the coroner one or more " coroner's " physicians, whose duty it is to make all medico-legal examinations, or a police magistrate or some such official has the power to appoint a physician to conduct the same. It is obvious that the more attention any one physician gives to this kind of professional work, the better qualified will he be for performing it; in Philadelphia the coroner usually appoints one physician as coroner's physician, though frequently he is allowed one or more assistants.

The compensation of the coroner's physician and assistants might either be by the fee system or by salary. The latter is much preferable, for, if the emolument of the office depends upon the number of post-mortem examinations made, these examinations might be increased needlessly. At the present time in this city the coroner's physician and assistant are salaried. Apart, however, from the case of the regularly appointed and salaried coroner's physician, any physician may be called upon by the Commonwealth or the defendant, in murder cases, for example, to give testimony. It is not only desirable, but most important under such circumstances, that if the physician agrees to give his time to the Commonwealth or the defense, the matter of compensation should be first definitely fixed. If a physician be subpœnaed as an ordinary witness, which summons he must obey, and, having given his evidence in court, the Commonwealth or the defense endeavors to obtain an expert expression of opinion upon the facts testified to in addition to the testimony as to the mere facts themselves, the physician is justified in refusing to answer. If, for example, a physician happened to see a man stabbed, and is subpœnaed as an ordinary witness to testify as to the facts, he must answer questions bearing directly upon such facts as he observed. But should the judge, prosecuting attorney, or defense ask a physician who has been so subpœnaed strictly professional questions which an ordinary witness, such as a laboring man, could not possibly answer, and which he alone can answer on account of his being specially qualified, the physician in justice to himself should refuse to answer them. The court has no more right to take advantage of the physician's professional knowledge and skill in extorting evidence without proper compensation than it would have to take his property; his knowledge is his property, his capital.* While in a general way it is always proper that every law-abiding citizen should contribute to the Commonwealth anything that lies in his power, whatever his profession may be, by which the ends of justice will be attained, it is only right that he should be sufficiently compensated by the Commonwealth for so doing.

* *Vide* Webb *vs.* Page: 1st Carrington and Kerwin's "Nisi Prius Reports," p. 23.

Relations of the Medical Profession to the Coroner.—

"The crowner hath sate on her and finds it Christian burial.
 But is this law?
 Ay, marry is't
 Crowner's-quest law."

In cases of persons dying from violence, or after an illness of less than twenty-four hours, no physician having been in attendance within said time, or that there were suspicious circumstances connected with the case, the coroner is notified by the attending physician, members of the family, or some one interested in the case. As there is some difference of opinion among physicians and lawyers as to the interpretation of the law bearing upon such cases, it is well that the law should be stated. By the Act of Assembly, March 22, 1867, it is provided: "That it shall be the duty of the coroner of the city and county of Philadelphia to hold an inquest on the body of any deceased person who shall have died a violent death, or whose death shall be sudden; provided, that such sudden death be after an illness of less than twenty-four hours, and that no regular practising physician shall have been in attendance within said time, or that suspicious circumstances shall render the same necessary; which said suspicions shall first be sworn to by one or more citizens of said city." Such being the law, the attending physician may say that, while in cases of death from violence or occurring under suspicious circumstances, it is undoubtedly his duty to notify the coroner, this law cannot be so interpreted as to compel him to notify the coroner in cases of death from chronic disease, even though he may not have been in attendance within twenty-four hours of death.

2

Let us suppose that a physician, in accordance with that interpretation of the law, signs a death-certificate, assigning some chronic disease as the cause of death, not having seen the patient for several days, or weeks perhaps, before death. It is not impossible that in such a case suspicions might be aroused after burial, the body might be exhumed, and a post-mortem examination might reveal poison as the true cause of death. An attending physician, under these circumstances, would certainly be subpœnaed to appear before the coroner to explain his action, even though he were not held for criminal prosecution.

It may be urged, however, if the attending physician notifies the coroner in such cases, that the coroner will order a post-mortem examination to be made, will hold an inquest, bringing his jury to the house, thereby needlessly annoying the family of the deceased and outraging their feelings. As a matter of fact, however, there is no necessity that the family should be annoyed in the slightest degree. The coroner, being notified, will either authorize the attending physician to sign the certificate, or send his physician to the house to simply inspect the body, and possibly to ascertain if the family and friends of the deceased are entirely satisfied as to the cause of death.

On the other hand, let us suppose that the attending physician does not notify the coroner in a case of death from chronic disease where he has not been in attendance within a period of twenty-four hours, and that the attention of the coroner is called to the fact that the life of the deceased was heavily insured, or that the insurance company objects to the payment of the premiums for some reason. Under such circumstances the coroner is obliged to have the body exhumed, a post-mortem examination made, the attending physician and members of the family of deceased perhaps subpœnaed to appear at his office, the inquest only proving that the true cause of death was such as was first assigned in the death-certificate. All such trouble and annoyance can be avoided in such cases by simply notifying the coroner. However, therefore, the law bearing on such cases may be interpreted, why should the attending physician assume any responsibility, and risk future trouble when there is an official regularly appointed for the investigation of such cases?

It is sometimes also held by physicians that the law cannot compel the attending physician to notify the coroner in a case of death from violence, if death be delayed several months or years. Such an opinion, however, is a misinterpretation of the law, and would not be sustained, since it is distinctly stated in the act, without qualification that the coroner shall hold an inquest " on the body of any deceased person who shall have died a violent death." Indeed, even if the attending physician were fully satisfied that the cause of death could not be even remotely traced to some act of violence or injury suffered by the deceased years before death, it would be advisable for him to notify the coroner to relieve himself of any responsibility, in the view of a suit for damages possibly being instituted.

Whatever views physicians may hold as to the propriety of the law regulating the conduct of the coroner, it is well for them to realize the authority enjoyed by that official, at least in this Commonwealth, before entering into any conflict with him. The office is an exceedingly old one, having been in existence hundreds of years, antedating that of any of the judges of our courts.

> " At sessions ther was he lord and sire;
> Ful often time he was knight of the shire.
> A shereve hadde he ben and a coronour
> Was no where swiche a worthy vavasour. ''

He can subpœna any one to his office at any hour of the day, and commit for contempt. The coroner has an enormous amount of authority, if he chooses to exercise it, and if he abuses it can give those with whom he comes in official contact endless trouble and annoyance. Indeed, so true is this that the office has been abolished in many places. Such being the case, so long as the office exists, the author would recommend to physicians to "keep o' the windy side of the law" and to notify the coroner in all doubtful cases involving his jurisdiction, thereby saving themselves much annoyance, trouble, and loss of time.

CHAPTER II.

Signs of Death—Cessation of Circulation and Respiration—Loss of Sensibility of the Eyes to Light—Ashy Pallor—Loss of Heat—Rigor Mortis—Cadaveric Spasm—Suggillation—Putrefaction—Conversion of Bodies into Adipocere—Length of Time Elapsing Since Death—Symptoms and Post-mortem Appearances of Death from Diseases of Brain, Heart, and Lungs—Presumption of Death—Presumption of Survivorship.

It is frequently stated that persons have been buried alive, or we hear of individuals having been aroused with great difficulty from a state of trance or catalepsy, premature burial being thereby fortunately prevented. If the slightest doubt prevails as to whether a person is dead, a physician should certainly not give a death-certificate, still less contemplate opening the body. While there is no doubt that all accounts of persons being buried alive are very much exaggerated, nevertheless, as these statements may not be entirely without foundation, it is most important that the physician should be familiar with the signs of death. There are a number of signs by which a living body can be distinguished from a dead body.

Cessation of Circulation and Respiration.—The continuous cessation of the circulation and respiration may be regarded unequivocally as indicating death.* It is impossible to conceive of a human being living for any length of time—half an hour, for example—if the heart has ceased to beat or the lungs to expand and contract during that

* Tidy, Charles Meymott: "Legal Medicine," London, 1882, part I, pp. 32, 36.

21

period. Not infrequently, however, it is very difficult to determine positively whether the heart is beating or not, or to state positively that respiration has entirely ceased. It is well known that certain animals, like the marmot, are in the habit, during the winter months, of hibernating. This condition is one of deep and prolonged sleep, the animal taking no food during that period, living upon itself. The beats of the heart, from being under ordinary circumstances 80 to 90 per minute, are reduced to 8 or 9. The respirations are so infrequent, and follow each other at such long intervals, that the most experienced and careful observer will often find it difficult to convince himself that the blood is really circulating, and that the animal is breathing. Nevertheless, such is the case, for, toward the spring, with the taking of food the creature begins to show evidence of returning vitality. The heart increases in the strength and number of its beats, the respiration increases in its frequency and force, and with the spring once well set in the normal activity of the animal is re-established.

A similar condition is presented, to a certain extent, in the case of human beings in a state of trance or catalepsy, of syncope and asphyxia, and in patients who have been suffering from prolonged disease of a low typhoid state. Under such circumstances the heart often beats so slowly and infrequently, the respiratory movements of the chest are so slight, that the most careful and closest inspection is required to determine whether the patient is alive. In such cases, however, if a ligature be bound around one of the fingers, the part between the ligature and the end of the finger, if the blood is still circulating, will become a deep red or purple in color, through the congestion due to the arrest of the circulation at that point. But no such change will be observed if life is extinct. Further, if respiration has not entirely ceased, by placing a mirror in front of the mouth the watery vapor exhaled can usually be detected through its condensing as a slight cloud upon the glass. The presence of such a cloud, however faint, is a proof that the person is still living.

Loss of sensibility of the eyes to light is a characteristic sign of death. When a lighted candle is brought near to the eye, the pupil contracts, and as it is removed from the eye the pupil dilates. This change in the size of the pupil may be regarded as a characteristic of vitality; for, though the phenomenon may occur within a few hours after death, the muscular fibers of the iris, sooner or later, like all muscular fibers, lose their power of contractility. Atropia, also, on account of its effect in dilating, and Calabar bean, by reason of its effect in contracting the pupil, may be used as determining whether life is extinct.

The **ashy pallor** of the body may be regarded as a sign of death, though not a characteristic one, since it is not present in death from all diseases, as in a person dying, for instance, from jaundice or from yellow fever.

Loss of Heat.—One of the most remarkable of vital phenomena is the power man possesses of maintaining, through chemical processes, the temperature of his body at about 98.6° F. whatever be the character of the surroundings, whether the region be tropic or arctic, whether the season be winter or summer. After death, however, the body, through radiation, conduction, convection, loses heat, and at first very quickly. During the first three hours after death the body may lose perhaps as much as four degrees per hour. The temperature then progressively falls at the rate of a degree and a half an hour until, within between fifteen and twenty-four hours after death, it is that of the surrounding atmosphere.*

In some cases, however, the cooling of the body may be completed within from two to seven hours after death, while in others the period may be extended to upward of four days. Thus, in the well-known Lowestoft case, in which three children were drowned by the mother placing their heads in a pail of water, the bodies were found perfectly cold after an expiration of six and a half hours. On the other hand, cases have been reported in which the body retained its heat so long after death as to render it doubtful whether death had really taken place.

Loss of heat is a characteristic sign of death, but there are certain conditions which influence the rate at which the body cools. Bodies that are thin and emaciated cool more quickly than fat ones, fat being a non-conductor. The bodies of young children lose heat more rapidly than those of adults, and the bodies of old people more rapidly than those of individuals in the prime of life. A body that is exposed to the air will lose its heat more quickly than when it is inclosed, and a body unclothed will lose heat more quickly than if it were clothed. If the room in which a dead body is lying be large and airy, the heat will be given off more rapidly than if the room be a small, close, and confined one. A body immersed in water loses its heat more rapidly than when it is exposed to the air.

It should be mentioned in this connection that in per-

* Taylor and Wilks: "Guy's Hospital Reports," third series, vol. IX, October, 1863, p. 180; Niderkorn: "Rigidité cadaverique chez l'Homme," Paris, 1872; Burman: "Edinburgh Medical Journal," vol. XXV, 1880, p. 993; Goodhart: "British Medical Journal," 1874, p. 303; "Guy's Hospital Reports," 1870, p. 365.

sons dying from yellow fever, smallpox, tetanus, cholera, and from some other acute diseases, and in animals, such as cats and dogs, poisoned by strychnia, there often occurs a rise instead of a fall of temperature. The cause of this increase of temperature, amounting in certain instances to as much as 9° F., is not yet understood.

When the various conditions that modify the rate at which the body cools after death are taken into consideration, it becomes evident that the medical examiner should express himself most cautiously in regard to the time that has elapsed since death or the cause of the same.

Rigor mortis (cadaveric rigidity), or the stiffening of the muscles throughout the body, is a characteristic sign of death. While usually appearing within three to six hours after death, rigor mortis may set in before the heart has ccased to beat or may be delayed until fifteen to twenty hours. It may last only a few moments, or from twenty-four to forty-eight hours, or even weeks. The variations in time of its appearance and duration appear to depend upon the previous condition of the body, any cause that depresses or exhausts muscular irritability favoring its early appearance. Thus, rigor mortis sets in early in the cases of soldiers killed late in battle, of persons dying of lingering, exhaustive fevers, of phthisis, cholera, convulsions, of animals overdriven, etc. On the other hand, rigor mortis sets in late in cases of persons dying in full muscular vigor, as in death from decapitation, apoplexy, hemorrhage, wounds of the heart, medulla, etc. It may be stated as a general rule that when rigor mortis sets in early it soon passes away, as in cases of narcotic poisoning. On the other hand, if it sets in late it lasts long, in cases of death from suffocation it not appearing maybe until sixteen hours after death, and persisting for several days. In cases of strychnia-poisoning, however, though the rigor sets in early, it persists for a long time.

It is often asserted that in death from electricity, and in the case of animals hunted to death, rigor mortis does not occur. This statement is erroneous, inasmuch as rigor mortis is the sequence of death from any cause. In the instances just mentioned the rigor sets in so early and passes off so quickly as to readily escape observation.

The order in which the muscles pass into the condition of rigor mortis is a very definite one. The muscles of the eye first become rigid; then successively the muscles of the neck, chest, upper extremities, and finally the muscles of the lower extremities. It should be mentioned in this connection, however, that considerable difference of opinion has prevailed among those * who have especially studied the phenomena of rigor mortis as to the exact order in which the different parts of the body pass into that condition, as well as the time of its appearance and duration. Rigor mortis disappears in the same order; that is, the muscles of the neck relax first. The muscles of the extremities may still be rigid, even though the remaining muscles are relaxed. After the rigor mortis has entirely passed off the general pliancy of the body is restored, and decomposition at once begins. Rigor mortis is due to the coagulation of myosin, differing in this respect from ordinary muscular contraction.

* Nysten: "Récherches de Physiologie et de Chimie pathologiques, etc.," p. 384; Sommer: "De Signis Mortem Humanis Absolutem ante Putredinis Accessum Indicantibus," Hayniæ, 1833; "Particula Posterior Caput Octavium," p. 185; Larcher: "Archives des Générales Médecine," vol. i, 1862, p. 685; Maschka: "Handbuch der gerichtlichen Medicin," dritter Band, Tübingen, 1882.

Cadaveric spasm (spasmodic rigidity), or the spasm often occurring at the moment of death,[*] in the case of persons who have died from sudden or violent deaths, though resembling rigor mortis, and sooner or later passing into that condition, is not necessarily identical with it. Cadaveric spasm, occurring in cases of violent or sudden death, appears to be due to all the vital energy having been concentrated in the one final muscular effort, and not at all to coagulation of the myosin of the muscle. Thus, the soldier may be found dead on the field of battle grasping his musket in the act of taking aim, the suicide or murdered person clutching the weapon he held in his hand the moment before death, the weapons in such cases being often grasped with such firmness that after death it requires considerable force to remove them.

Such facts, as we shall see hereafter, have an important practical bearing from a medico-legal point of view. Thus, if a pistol or razor be found firmly grasped in the hand of a dead person, it would be a strong presumption, apart from any other consideration, that it was a case of suicide, since such a condition cannot be successfully imitated by a murderer.

Suggillation.—In connection with the signs of death, the conditions known as *cadaveric lividity*, or suggillation, may appropriately be mentioned. It is the result of the settling of blood in the capillaries, and gives rise to violet-colored or livid patches, which, while at first isolated, afterward coalesce. Such discolorations are observed in the most dependent parts of the body, such as the back, under surface of the neck, calves of the legs, etc. When

---

[*] Brinton: "American Journal of Medical Science," Jan., 1870; Ogston: "British and Foreign Medical Review," April, 1857, p. 303.

occurring in the lungs and other internal organs, cadaveric lividity is known as hypostatic congestion. Cadaveric lividity is sometimes mistaken for a bruise. The latter condition can, however, readily be distinguished from cadaveric lividity, since, if a bruise be divided by a scalpel, either effused blood or a clot will be found.

Putrefaction, or the decomposition of nitrogenous substances by certain bacteria, with the development of gaseous, foul-smelling products, is usually regarded as the most positive sign of death.* While the phenomena of putrefaction are undoubtedly due to the presence of bacteria, the products of the decomposition of the albuminous substances being subsequently modified by the oxidizing action of the air, the free access of which affords the most favorable condition for the introduction of the bacteria, nevertheless, the rapidity of the process will be greatly influenced, not only by the amount of moisture present in the atmosphere and by the temperature of the latter, but also by the age, sex, condition of the body, and cause of death, as well as by the period, place, and mode of burial. Putrefaction, for example, is arrested in the presence of perfectly dry air. Thus, in the sandy deserts of Arabia and Africa a dead body, losing rapidly its fluids, dries up and mummifies, while bodies buried naked or but very little clothed, in wooden coffins, in shallow graves to which the air ordinarily has access, putrefy rapidly. The influence of temperature in promoting or retarding putrefaction is well shown by the fact that bodies putrefy more rapidly in summer than in winter. Indeed, putrefaction is entirely arrested at a temperature of 32° F., bodies of men and

* Flügge, Dr. C.: "Micro-organisms," translated by W. W. Cheyne, London, 1890, p. 608.

animals buried in ice for nearly a hundred years having been found in a state of perfect preservation after exhumation. Thus, for example, the body of Prince Menschikoff, banished to Siberia by Peter the Great, was found, on exhumation from frozen soil, but little changed, though it had been buried for ninety-two years. The corpses preserved at the hospice of Mont St. Bernard, where the temperature is usually below the freezing-point, are recognizable after many years. It is well known that the flesh of a mammoth exposed through the thawing of the ice on the banks of the Lena River in Siberia was in such an excellent state of preservation that it was eagerly devoured by dogs, wolves, bears, etc.

The temperature most favorable to putrefaction appears to be between 70° and 100° F., a temperature of 212° F. arresting it.

Other things equal, the bodies of children putrefy more rapidly than those of adults and of aged persons, and the bodies of the aged more rapidly than those of adults. Putrefaction appears to be more rapid in women than in men. The rapidity with which bodies putrefy is also influenced by the condition of the body and the causes of death. Thus, fat and flabby bodies, those of new-born children, and of women dying in childbirth, putrefy rapidly, probably on account of the amount of fluid present in the body under such circumstances. The bodies of persons dying from exhaustive diseases, such as typhus fever, or from injuries involving the bruising and mangling of the bodies, or from poisonous gases like carbonic oxid, etc., undergo putrefaction quickly. Putrefaction is retarded, on the other hand, in cases of death from alcohol, phosphorus, arsenic, and certain narcotic poisons. Putrefaction is hastened or retarded according to the period of the year at which death occurs, and the place and mode of burial. Thus, bodies putrefy more quickly in summer than in winter. Putrefaction takes place more rapidly in air than in water; more rapidly in water than in earth. Indeed, according to Casper,* the degree of putrefaction present in a body after lying in the open air for one week corresponds to that found in a body after lying in water two weeks, or after burial in the earth in the usual manner eight weeks. Three bodies will, therefore, exhibit *caet par* about the same degree of putrescence of which one shall have been lying in an open field for one week, a second in water for two weeks, and a third after burial in a coffin in the usual manner eight weeks. Putrefaction goes on rapidly in low, moist, swampy regions, slowly in dry, elevated ones. The deeper a body is buried and the better it is protected from the air by clothes or coffin, the slower the putrefaction. Notwithstanding what has just been stated in regard to the various conditions influencing the progress of putrefaction, as it is well known that the decomposition of bodies of the same general character buried in the same kind of coffins and graves varies very considerably, there must be other conditions, not so well understood in their effects as those just mentioned, that are also concerned in the production of putrefaction.

Inasmuch as putrefaction is influenced by so many conditions, it is impossible to state exactly when it will first appear or the length of time before a body will entirely be decomposed. As a general rule,† it may be said, in the case

---

* Casper: "Handbook of the Practice of Forensic Medicine," 4 vols., London, 1861, vol. i, p. 37.

† Casper: *op. cit.*, vol. i, pp. 39, 40.

of bodies exposed to the open air, that within a period after death of from one to three days in summer, and three to six days in winter, there appears a greenish or greenish-yellow spot upon the abdomen about three inches in diameter, accompanied by the peculiar odor of putrefaction. The eyeball at the same time becomes soft and yielding. During the next succeeding few days—three to five—this greenish discoloration spreads over the body in coalescing spots.

In about eight to ten days the chest and abdomen become distended and swollen with the gases which in the mean time develop. The sphincter ani becomes relaxed, and reddish streaks appear along the course of the blood-vessels. Fourteen to twenty days after death the epidermis is raised here and there in blisters about the size of a walnut, which shortly break. Innumerable maggots have made their appearance, and the nails have loosened. The development of gases continuing, the thorax and abdomen become enormously distended. The penis is very much swollen and shapeless, and the scrotum is enlarged, in some cases, to the size of a child's head. The hairs of the head are loose and can readily be pulled out. Within a period of from four to six months the walls of the body-cavities burst open, discharging their contents. The brain runs out, and the orbital cavities are empty. All the soft parts have either become pulpy or have disappeared. The softened flesh falls away from the bones, the skeleton thereby becoming exposed. The sexes finally become indistinguishable, unless a uterus is recognizable or the pubic hair or its mode of growth can be distinguished, the hair, as is well known, being limited to the mons veneris in the female, but extending upward to the navel in the male sex.

As a general rule, the order in which the internal organs putrefy is quite a regular one. Inferences from their condition as to the time elapsing since death are far more trustworthy, therefore, than those based upon an examination of the body externally. The first part of the body to putrefy internally is the mucous membrane of the larynx and trachea, which becomes a dirty red in color, at the same time that the abdomen becomes greenish externally, as just described. In young infants the next organ to decompose is the brain. Then follow the stomach and intestines. In this connection it should be mentioned that the ordinary post-mortem redness of the mucous membrane of the stomach often resembles so closely that due to poisoning that the superficial examiner might readily be deceived and attribute such a condition to poison having been taken. Further, the medical examiner should always be on his guard lest he mistake for putrefaction that condition of the stomach due to post-mortem digestion, it being well known since the time of John Hunter * that the stomach, and more particularly its cardiac portion, is often after death digested by its own gastric juice. The spleen, omentum and mesentery, and liver, if healthy at time of death, may resist putrefaction for several weeks. The brain in the adult, though a soft structure, does not usually putrefy before the fourth or fifth week. The next organs to putrefy are usually the heart and lungs. Then follow the kidneys, esophagus, pancreas, diaphragm, and arteries. The last organ to decompose is the uterus, which in certain cases has been recognized even seven months after death.

* "Philosophical Transactions," London, 1772, p. 447.

As an illustration of the practical importance of this fact may be mentioned the celebrated case described by Casper,[*] in which the remains of a human being were discovered in a privy in a more advanced state of putrefaction than had hitherto been noticed by that observer, and yet the uterus was found still perfectly recognizable and in such a good state of preservation as to enable him to state positively that the deceased could not have been pregnant at the time of her death. By this important testimony the innocence of a man of irreproachable character was established who had been falsely accused of seducing a servant girl in his employ, of getting her with child, and, tiring of her, murdering her and then throwing her into the privy—simply because the girl had disappeared.

Conversion into Adipocere.—Under certain circumstances a dead body, instead of undergoing putrefaction in the ordinary manner, is converted into the substance known as "adipocere," so called on account of its general resemblance to a combination of fat and wax.[†] Adipocere, being chemically either ammonium or calcium stearate or oleate, is probably produced through the combination of a fatty acid of the fat with the ammonium resulting from the decomposition of the nitrogenous tissues, the ammonium being often replaced afterward by calcium. The formation of adipocere being, therefore, a saponification, the presence of water, as might be expected, is essential to its production. Dead bodies are, therefore, converted into adipocere only in graves containing water, or in wet or at

[*] Casper: *op. cit.*, vol. I, p. 53

[†] Fourcroy: "Annales de Chimie," tome v, 1790, p. 154; tome VII, p. 17; Chevreul: *ibid.*, tome xcv, p. 5; Orfila et Lesueur: "Traité des Exhumations juridiques," tome I, Paris, 1831, p. 351; Schauenstein in Maschka, Band III, S. 445.

3

least very moist soil. Inasmuch as dead bodies lying in water for any length of time may be converted into adipocere, it becomes a matter of importance to determine the length of time required for such conversion, since it will enable the medical examiner to state, in a general way at least, how long the body has been lying in the water when it was found. As the result of observations and experiments it may be said that, on the average, the body of a new-born child will be changed into adipocere after remaining in water between five and six weeks. An adult body requires, for complete conversion into adipocere one year if immersed in water, and three years or more if buried in wet earth.*

Length of Time Elapsing Since Death.—Having described in a general way the signs of death, there still remains for consideration the question as to the medical examiner being enabled from such signs alone to determine positively the length of time which has elapsed since death. That it is highly important that the medical examiner should be able to give such testimony has been well shown in cases of murder, such as those in which the defendant endeavored to prove an alibi, and the prosecution, by medical testimony, that the wounds causing death were not inflicted during the period that the defendant claimed he was absent.

It must be admitted, however, notwithstanding the verdict of guilty often rendered in such cases based upon that kind of evidence, that any estimate as to the length of time elapsing since death based upon post-mortem examination alone can only be approximative. In a general way, therefore, it can only be stated, in the case of the body being

* Devergie: "Médecine légale," tome I, Paris, p. 97.

unburied and exposed to the atmosphere, that if the body is only slightly cold and the jaws beginning to stiffen, the eyes glazed and the eyeball sunken, death has occurred within a period of from fifteen minutes to four hours. If, however, the entire body be cold and rigid, the abdomen has turned green and the odor of putrefaction is perceptible, the body is cold and pliant, and there is cadaveric lividity, the rigor mortis having passed away, death has taken place within from one to three days in summer and from three to six days in winter. If greenish-brown stains and dark red lines are found extending more or less over a greenish-yellow body, together with relaxation of the sphincter ani muscle, then death has occurred within a period of from eight to ten days in summer, ten to twenty days in winter. If the entire body is green, the chest and abdomen enormously distended, if open blisters are found over the skin, and maggots in the muscles, the nails falling out, the color of the eyes unrecognizable, then death has occurred within a period of from two to three weeks in summer, of from four to six weeks in winter. If the contents of the chest and abdomen have been discharged, some of the bones bare, the orbital cavities empty, death has taken place within a period of from four to six months.

Symptoms and Post-mortem Appearances of Death from Diseases of the Brain, Heart, and Lungs.—Whatever be the remote cause of death in any particular instance, whether it be due to disease, injury, wounds, or fractures, it may be referred approximately, at least, to an arrest of the action of the brain, heart, or lungs. In order to be able to determine the cause of death, the medical examiner should be familiar with the symptoms and post-mortem appearances of death as due to the three causes just mentioned.

The symptoms of death beginning at the brain, or coma, are stupor, insensibility to external impressions, loss of consciousness; slow, stertorous, irregular breathing; the respiration and circulation ceasing as the medulla becomes affected. The post-mortem appearances presented in the case of death beginning at the brain are effusion of blood into the cavities, due to apoplexy, rupture of the blood-vessels from fracture of the skull, embolism, abscess, congestion, and compression. Death beginning at the heart, or syncope, may be due to a deficiency in the quantity of the blood, or anæmia; or in the quality, or asthenia. Death from anæmia may be caused by rupture of an aneurysm, or from a uterine hemorrhage, or from a division of a large vessel, like the carotid artery. The symptoms of such conditions are paleness, lividity of lips, dimness of vision, vertigo, slow, fluttering, weak pulse, ringing in the ears, hallucination, with more or less delirium and nausea and loss of brain power. On post-mortem examination the heart is usually found contracted and empty, especially if the latter is examined shortly after death.

Death due to the asthenic condition occurs in fatty degeneration of the heart, in exhaustive diseases of any kind, starvation, and in poisoning from prussic acid. The symptoms in such cases are cold hands and feet, lividity of lips, nose, and extremities, great muscular weakness, feeble pulse, senses and intelligence retained usually till the last. After death the heart is found contracted, or its cavities are dilated and flabby, and contain blood.

Death beginning at the lungs, or asphyxia, is caused by mechanical obstacles, such as foreign bodies in the air-passages. Respiration may be arrested by spasm of the glottis, due to nervous excitement, or by paralysis of the respiratory muscles. The symptoms of a person dying from asphyxia are lividity of the face, great dyspnœa, vertigo, loss of consciousness, and convulsions. In death from asphyxia the venous system and the right side of the heart and lungs are found filled with dark blood. The left side of the heart and the arterial system, if rigor mortis has set in, are, however, usually found empty.

Whatever may be the remote cause of death, the immediate cause is, then, to be looked for in the brain, heart, or lungs. A characteristic set of symptoms precedes death, accompanied by characteristic post-mortem appearances in most cases. The medical examiner should usually be able, therefore, to determine at least the approximate cause of death. It sometimes happens, however, that there is no history of the case and, notwithstanding the fact that a most careful post-mortem examination has been made, the cause of death cannot be positively determined. Under such circumstances it may be supposed that there has been possibly sudden stoppage of the heart through reflex nervous inhibition, as occurs in persons who have drunk cold water when in an overheated condition, or as the result of some violent emotion. In such cases no post-mortem lesion of any kind may be found. It can only be said then that death may be supposed to have been due to some nervous influence. It is not worth while, however, for the medical examiner to guess or speculate about the cause of death. The most prudent course to pursue in such cases, in reply to any questions, is to admit that the cause of death cannot be stated.

Presumption of Death.—It not infrequently happens that a person leaves his home and is not heard of for many continuous years, perhaps never again. The law presuming such a person to be dead, the executor is justified in settling the estate. The length of time usually assumed legally as warranting the presumption of death is seven years from the time the person was last seen or heard of.* A woman who had not heard of her husband for that number of years might marry again, therefore, without rendering herself liable to the charge of bigamy, even if it were afterward shown that the first husband was living at the time of the second marriage. In cases where property is inherited, and in life-insurance cases, so long a time as seven years is not usually considered necessary by the courts, settlements being often made in two years of the period within which the person was presumed to have died. The presumption of death is usually determined by a jury on the general evidence submitted.

Under certain circumstances, however, as in cases where the person presumed to be dead was suffering from some disease at the time last seen or heard of, medical testimony would be taken as to the probable issue in such a case.

Presumption of Survivorship.—When several persons, members of the same family, for example, are lost at sea or are burned up in a fire, etc., the law of the present day, like the old Roman law, usually assumes that they perished together. Not infrequently, however, in such cases efforts are made, by relatives interested in the disposition of an estate thus left, to prove by medical testimony that some one member of the family survived the others, and that such a one was the heir at law. Suppose that the persons dying were father and son, and that the son survived the father, even though it were for a moment, his

* Beck, J. B.: "Medical Jurisprudence," Philadelphia, 1860, vol. i, p. 643; Tidy: *op. cit.*, part i, p. 381.

wife would inherit—"shall have dower for the lands descended the instant the father died"; or, for example, that two persons were related to each other as testator and legatee, and that the latter should die first; the legacy would then lapse. If, however, the legatee survived the testator, then his heirs would inherit. A husband inherits from his wife if their child survives the death of the mother, even for only a moment—" as tenant by curtesy."*

While no positive statements can be made by the medical examiner in such cases, there are, nevertheless, certain general probabilities that should be taken into consideration. Thus, for example, if a number of persons of different ages perish together, it would be a fair presumption that the very old and very young, other things being equal, would not survive as long as those of middle age. In the case of a man and woman being drowned, it is to be presumed that, on account of greater physical strength, the man survived longer than the woman. On the other hand, in cases of death from carbonic acid poisoning, women appear to survive longer than men (the proportion being as high, perhaps, as five to four, women as a rule consuming less oxygen than men), require less air, and will live, therefore, longer in an imperfectly ventilated room or one containing noxious gases.

Young people and old persons appear to succumb more quickly to the effects of cold than those of middle age. The latter, however, do not resist the effects of heat so well as the former. As regards the effects of cold and heat upon the human system, more particularly in reference to questions of survivorship, the general physical condition, the

* Blackstone: " Commentaries," London, 1829, vol. II, p. 126.

kind of clothing, the extent to which alcohol has been indulged in, would have to be taken into consideration.

It is well known that the aged can do without food better than adults, and adults better than the young, the latter needing food not only for the repair of the tissues and the liberation of energy, but for growth. In cases of death from starvation the presumption would be, therefore, in favor of the aged surviving, rather than the adult or the young. In case of two persons dying of starvation, one fat, the other emaciated, the presumption would be that the fat person would live longer than the emaciated one, the former having a greater supply of fat to draw upon to maintain life than the latter, nine-tenths of the fat of the body disappearing in a death from starvation.

In the case of mother and child dying in child-bed, in the absence of witnesses it is usually assumed that the mother survived the child, the *prima facie* probability being that the child was stillborn and that the mother would be, under ordinary circumstances, unable to minister to the child. Such an opinion would be still further confirmed if there were evidences of a difficult labor, of the child being a large one, and absence of the signs of respiration.

In the event of the death of several persons from wounds, it has been held, for example, by Casper and Liman, that if three individuals died respectively from a bayonet wound of the heart, a gunshot wound opening the jugular vein, and a saber cut of the head, death would take place in the three instances in the above order.* While under ordinary circumstances such presumption would be a reasonable one, nevertheless it might be otherwise, since a soldier upon

* Wharton and Stillé: "Medical Jurisprudence," Phila., 1884, vol. III, p. 576.

whom the author made a post-mortem examination, lived four hours after a penetrating bayonet wound of the heart, the fatal hemorrhage having been delayed apparently by a blood-clot, whereas in the case of a man who died from rupture of the internal jugular vein, as shown by the author on post-mortem examination, death occurred within a few seconds of the rupture.

In the recent case of the Young Women's Christian Home, appellant, *vs.* John L. French, administrator of Eugene Rhodes, deceased (appeals from the Court of Appeals of the District of Columbia), tried during the October term, 1902, of the Supreme Court of the United States, it was shown that Mrs. Sophia Rhodes, a widow, and her son, Eugene, her only child, perished at sea, on the occasion of the sinking of the steamer "Elbe," January 30, 1895. The question at once arose, Which of the two—mother or son—survived, at least temporarily? If the son survived the mother, the next of kin of the son would inherit; whereas, if the mother survived the son, or the two died simultaneously, the Young Women's Christian Home would inherit, that being clearly the intention of the testatrix as expressed in her will, in the event of her surviving her husband and son. The opinion of the Court, as delivered by Mr. Chief Justice Fuller, was as follows:

"The rule is that there is no presumption of survivorship in the case of persons who perish by a common disaster, in the absence of proof tending to show the order of dissolution, and that circumstances surrounding the calamity of the character appearing on this record are insufficient to create any presumption on which the courts can act. The question of actual survivorship is regarded as unascertainable, and descent and distribution take the same course as if the deaths had been simultaneous."

This opinion in regard to the question of survivorship is a most important one, since it is the first opinion of the kind, so far as known to the author, that has ever been delivered in the Supreme Court of the United States, and will be regarded, therefore, as a precedent probably for years to come.

In regard to those cases in which the time and date of death of one person are known, but those of the other are only presumed, the decision in regard to the question of survivorship must be entirely based upon the evidence. Thus, in the often-cited case of the loss of the steamer "Pulaski," in 1838, by explosion, through which a Mr. Ball and his wife lost their lives, it was decided by Chancellor Johnston that the wife survived the husband, upon the ground that the wife had been seen alive and heard calling her husband, whereas the husband was neither seen nor heard after the explosion. The case was appealed, but the above decision was reaffirmed.

CHAPTER III.

Autopsies—Corpus Delicti—Manner of Making Post-mortem Examinations in Medico-legal Cases—Identification of the Dead—Coroner's Inquest—Conduct of the Medical Witness in Court—Dying Declarations—Wills.

Autopsies.—In cases of sudden death, or death from violence, or death under suspicious circumstances, the coroner views the body, and if not satisfied as to the cause of death, directs his physician to make a post-mortem examination, the extent and thoroughness of which will depend entirely upon his discretion. It is essential that the results of the examination should be recorded at once in a book kept for that purpose, the examiner not waiting until he reaches his home, trusting to his memory for the facts. Neither should the record of the post-mortem examination made in one book at the time be transferred later to another book, since the objection may be made that the two records are not the same. It is needless to add that the coroner's physician should have his name and address distinctly written in his note-book, so that in case it is lost it may be advertised for, or the opportunity afforded for its return to its owner without delay.

Before beginning the post-mortem examination the place, the year, the day of the month, and the hour of the day should be recorded by the examiner.

Corpus Delicti.—The deceased must then be identified from their own personal knowledge, and not from hearsay, by two witnesses who knew the individual upon whom the post-mortem is to be made. It is not only important, but absolutely essential, that the corpus delicti—that is, the proof that the body upon which the autopsy is to be made is that of the person whose death the defendant is accused of being the cause—should be satisfactorily established. Thus, according to the Gothic constitution, it is insisted that before any fine can be exacted from the neighborhood for the slaughter of a man therein, *"de corpore delicti constare oportebat."* * The necessity of establishing the corpus delicti is emphasized by authorities on criminal law by such observations as: *"Diligenter cavendum est judici ne supplicium praecipitet antequam de crimine consteterit";* *"De corpore interfecti necesse est ut constet,"* etc.†

It is owing to the neglect of the observance of this precaution, the establishing of the corpus delicti, that innocent persons are convicted and executed and that guilty ones escape, the prosecution breaking down, failing entirely to make out its case. Among such cases may be mentioned those of the Frenchman who was convicted of the murder of a widow who subsequently returned to her home, having received no injury whatever; and of the two brothers Boorn, who were convicted of murder and who would have been executed had not their alleged victim fortunately reappeared. More remarkable still was the case of the three Trailor brothers, tried for the murder of a man named Fisher, on the occasion of which one of the brothers made under oath a confession stating exactly how the homicide had been committed, and which would have secured conviction, when, to the amazement of the court, Fisher, who

* Blackstone: *op. cit.,* vol. i, p. 348, note t.

† Wharton and Stillé: "Medical Jurisprudence," fourth edition, Philadelphia, 1884, vol. iii, p. 613.

was supposed to have been murdered, suddenly appeared. Extraordinary as it may seem, the confession was made by Trailor to cut the trial short, he supposing that it would end in his conviction and that of his brothers.

It may be appropriately mentioned in this connection that on the occasion of a murder trial in which the author gave testimony as a witness, although the corpus delicti had been established, as the name of the deceased was not the same as that in the indictment, the defense claimed that there was no evidence to show that the deceased upon whom the autopsy was made was the same person for whose murder the defendant was held. The contention being sustained by the Court, the defendant left the court a free man. It must be recognized, however, that in certain instances it would be impossible, from the very nature of the case, to obtain the body of the deceased to identify it. Thus, a man might be murdered at sea, as proved by eye-witnesses, and afterward thrown overboard, as in the case of the captain of the "Eolus," who was murdered by one of the sailors and whose body was never recovered. The body of a murdered person may be so completely destroyed by mechanical or chemical agents as to make it impossible to obtain any remains whatever for identification. Under such circumstances, even though no corpus delicti be proved, the guilty parties could be convicted if the evidence warranted such a verdict.

Manner of Making Post-mortem Examinations.—The corpus delicti having been established, if possible, the height of the deceased should then be determined, the examiner being always provided for this purpose with a tape-measure. This may become an important part of the testimony in certain cases, like that of murder, since it may be claimed that, the deceased being a taller man, and presumably heavier and stronger than the defendant, the murder was committed in self-defense. The body of the deceased should, therefore, be weighed. In a properly equipped morgue means are provided for this purpose. In their absence the weight of the body can at least be approximately estimated, and an idea can be obtained as to whether the deceased was strong, well built, muscular, or weak, sickly, emaciated. The temperature of the body and surrounding atmosphere should be noted; that of the morgue would usually be constant; but if the post-mortem examination be made elsewhere,—in a bar-room, in a yard, or in a field,—the temperature would be variable, according to circumstances, season of the year, etc. If the medical examiner be called upon to make an examination of a dead body in the place where it was first found, it is very important that all the surroundings should be most carefully and critically observed. If the dead body be found in a room, for example, its condition should be noted as to the position of the tables, chairs, china—whether the room was in order or confusion, the latter being probably the state in the case of there having been a struggle. The floor, walls, doors, windows, and furniture should be carefully examined for blood-stains or stains of any kind, footmarks. The condition of the clothing of the deceased should be noted as to whether it was cut or torn, etc. Indeed, no fact of any kind that could directly or indirectly aid in determining the cause of death, or lead to the arrest and conviction of the murderer, if murder has been committed, should fail to be recognized and recorded by the medical examiner.

A thorough examination having been made of the body

externally, and the situation, extent, and nature of the external injuries having been noted, if any such be present, the body should next be examined internally.* In making the internal examination it is best to begin with the head, except in cases of asphyxia, as in such cases, if the head is opened first, the blood is apt to run out of the right side of the heart. The scalp having been divided, and the two parts everted, the skull, after it has been examined carefully, should then be sawed through in such a manner that the calvaria † can be securely replaced. The dura mater, having been inspected, should then be divided and the condition of the arachnoid and pia mater be observed. The brain before removal should be examined as to congestion of its vessels, laceration of its substance, extravasation of blood, etc. After removal of the brain the base of the skull should be carefully examined for fractures. The

* Orth, Dr. Johannes: "Compend of Diagnosis in Pathological Anatomy, with Directions for Making Post-mortem Examinations," translated by F. E. Shattuck, M.D., and G. K. Sabine, M.D., New York, 1878; Virchow, Professor Rudolph: "Post-mortem Examinations with Special Reference to Medico-legal Practice," translated by J. P. Smith, M.D., Philadelphia, 1880; Casper: *op. cit.*, vol. I, p. 87.

† The word *calvarium*, often used synonymously with *calvaria*, does not appear, so far as known to the writer, to have been made use of by Latin authors. The neuter plural *calvaria* was used, however; for example, by Ennius in his description of certain marine animals: "Polypus Corcyræ, Calvaria purgina acarnæ, Purpura, Muriculi, Murex, dulces quoque echini" ("Enniariæ Poesis Reliquiæ," Lipseæ, 1854, p. 167). The acarnæ mentioned by Ennius are probably the fish referred to under that name by Aristotle and Pliny—the *Pagellus acharne* of Cuvier. Apuleius also uses the word *calvaria*, not, apparently, in the same sense in which that word is used by Ennius as parts of the Acarne, but as if the calvaria were distinct animals, the latter being referred to as "Marina calvaria" ("L. Apuleii, Opera Omnia," Lipseæ, 1842, pp. 520, 531).

condition of the brain should be noted as to its consistence, color, the existence of tumors, abscesses. The spinal column should next be opened through its whole extent, and the cord removed, and its condition noted. The thorax and abdomen should then be opened by making an incision extending from the root of the neck to the pubes, dividing the cartilages of the ribs and the sterno-clavicular ligaments, and reflecting the sternum. The heart, lungs, larynx, and trachea should be at once examined *in situ;* and after removal, parts of the organs should be preserved. The stomach, having been ligated at both the cardiac and the pyloric orifices, each orifice being secured by two ligatures, should then be removed by cutting between the two ligatures at each orifice, and placed in a clean glass jar. The intestines should be removed and preserved in a similar manner, though separately from the stomach. The condition of the liver, spleen, pancreas, kidneys, and urogenital apparatus should be noted, and portions of the organs preserved for microscopic examination if necessary.

As in murder trials the medical witness is not infrequently questioned in regard to the weight of the various organs of the human body, in connection with that of the organs found in the deceased, the following table is submitted as containing such information:

WEIGHTS OF ORGANS OF ADULTS.*

Heart, male,	11	oz.
Heart, female,	9	"
Brain, male,	49½	"
Brain, female,	44	"
Spinal cord,	1– 1¾	"
Liver,	50–60	"

* Woodman and Tidy: "A Handy Book of Forensic Medicine," etc., p. 11.

Pancreas,	$3\frac{1}{4}$– $3\frac{1}{2}$	oz.
Spleen,	5 – 7	"
Lungs (together), male,	45	"
Lungs (together), female,	32	"
Thyroid body,	1 – 2	"
Thymus at birth,	$\frac{1}{2}$	"
Kidneys (together),	9	"
Suprarenal capsules,	2	dr.
Prostate gland,	6	"
Testicles (together),	$\frac{3}{4}$– 1	oz.
Unimpregnated uterus,	7 –12	dr.

The post-mortem examination having been concluded, the calvaria should be replaced in position, the parts of the scalp inverted, and the latter, as well as the abdominal walls, brought together and securely sewed.

It need hardly be mentioned that in cases involving life or death the post-mortem examination should be thorough, lest the defense urge that the true cause of death be other than that alleged. In more than one case through such neglect has the prosecution failed to convict, owing to some organ not having been examined. Thus, in a well-known case where death appeared to be due to cerebro-spinal meningitis, rather than to tartar emetic poisoning, as alleged by the Commonwealth, nevertheless no examination of the spinal cord of the deceased was made. In another equally notorious case of alleged poisoning, while the symptoms indicated apoplexy and uræmia as the causes of death, the kidneys, as well as other organs, were never examined.* In both cases the prosecution failed to convict. and the verdict of acquittal was rather that of "not proven" than of "not guilty." On the other hand,

* Taylor, Alfred Swayne: "Manual of Medical Jurisprudence," eleventh American edition, by Clark Bell, Esq., Philadelphia, 1892, p. 23.

4

in another oft-quoted case, that of the man who was accused of beating his daughter to death for stealing, the real cause of death was found on thorough post-mortem examination to be, not the beating, but poison, the girl having taken arsenic with the hope of killing herself and thereby escaping the beating she knew she would receive on the detection of the theft.*

Identification.—Ordinarily the dead body submitted for medical examination is either entire or almost so. Not infrequently, however, the body has been purposely mutilated after death, by a murderer, for example, with the view of escaping detection, or as in cases of death from fire, explosions, railroad accidents. Under such circumstances, when often only parts of the body or bodies can be recovered for examination, the highest anatomical skill may be requisite for the identification of the remains or the determination of the cause of death. But little difficulty, however, should be experienced in determining, for example, whether the bones recovered be human or not, if the greater part of the skeleton, especially if parts of the skull, be submitted for examination. It is only when a bone or a fragment of a bone has been obtained, as from the ruins of a fire, that mistakes as to their true nature are likely to be made by the medical examiner. Inasmuch as the bones of the domestic animals have been frequently mistaken for those of man, even by physicians, if the examiner be in doubt as to the nature of a bone, it would be better for him to submit it to a comparative osteologist for determination, rather than to trust to his own judgment, unless specially qualified by previous osteologic studies to give an opinion on the subject.

* Wharton and Stillé: *op. cit.*, vol. III, p. 216.

As regards the skull more especially, there is usually no difficulty in determining whether it be a human one. The particular race, however, cannot always be indicated, for while there is no difficulty, for example, in distinguishing a

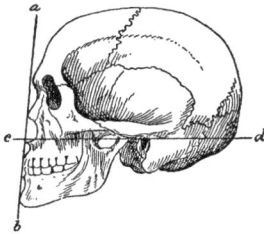

Fig. 1.—The facial angle of Camper. In European crania it usually does not exceed 80 degrees. *a, b, ·c, d,* Lines forming the facial angle.

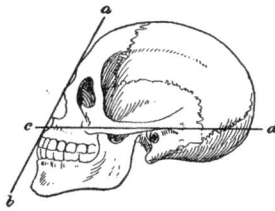

Fig. 2.—Facial angle of Camper ; in the negro, about 70 degrees. *a, b, c, d,* Lines forming the facial angle.

Caucasian skull (Fig. 1) from that of a typical negro (Fig. 2), it is not only difficult, but often impossible, to exactly identify the many forms of skull intermediate in character between the two. In the identification of human remains

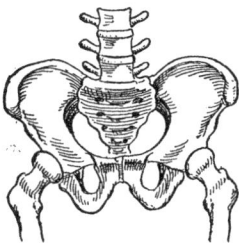

Fig. 3.—Male pelvis.

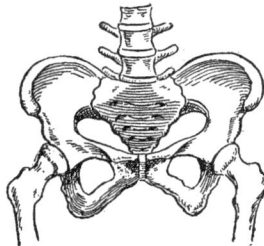

Fig. 4.—Female pelvis.

the sex, age, and stature are usually to be determined. Inasmuch as the skeleton of the male differs from that of the female as regards the size, weight, strength of the bones, in the relative development of the ridges and prominences serving for the attachment of the muscles, and more particularly in the size and shape of the pelvis (Figs. 3, 4), all of which peculiarities are fully described in works on anatomy, there is usually no difficulty, if the skeleton is entire, in determining whether it be that of a male or a female. If, however, a single bone or a fragment of a bone be submitted for an examination, it is often so difficult to determine the sex that no positive opinion should be expressed.

The age of a body can be approximately, at least, inferred from the development of the teeth and the extent of the ossification of the bones. It is important, therefore, that the medical examiner should be familiar with the period and order in which the teeth appear and the bones ossify. In the jaws of a child at full term there are usually found the rudiments of twenty primary and four secondary or permanent teeth, twenty-four teeth in all. The average date of the eruption or cutting of the primary or milk teeth is as follows: The four central incisors appear from five to eight months after birth; the four lateral incisors, from seven to ten months; the four anterior molars, from twelve to sixteen months; the four canines, from fourteen to twenty months; and the four posterior molars, from eighteen months to three years.* At a period of life varying between six and seven years the jaws contain forty-eight teeth—twenty milk teeth and twenty-eight permanent teeth situated behind the milk teeth, which they will replace as the former are shed. The order in which the permanent teeth appear is as follows: The four anterior molars appear at seven years; the four

* Bell, T.: "Anatomy, Physiology, and Diseases of the Teeth," 1837, pp. 66, 79.

central incisors, at eight years; the four lateral incisors, at nine years; the four anterior premolars, at ten years; the four posterior premolars, at eleven years; the four canines, at about twelve years; the four second molars, at about fourteen years;* the four posterior molars, at from eighteen to twenty-one years of age. As a general rule the teeth of the lower jaw appear first, but in this respect there are exceptions, as also in the order of the appearance of the teeth. It should be mentioned in this connection, also, that in cases of rickets the cutting of teeth is often delayed, while in syphilis it is premature.† In the latter

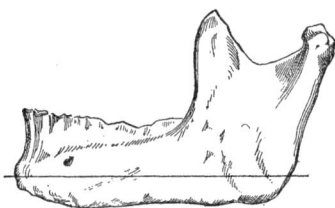

Fig. 5.—Lower jaw in the adult. Fig. 6.—Lower jaw in the aged.

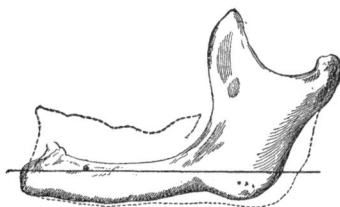

case the teeth have a notched appearance, and often crumble away. With the loss of the teeth and progressive absorption of the alveolar processes due to age, the lower jaw (Fig. 5) undergoes a marked change in the widening of the angle of its neck, and in the diminution of the width of its body (Fig. 6), imparting to the mouth the expression so characteristic of the aged.

* Saunders, Edwin : " The Teeth a Test of Age, Considered with Reference to the Factory Children," addressed to the members of both houses of Parliament; London, 1837, p. 42.

† Woodman and Tidy : " Handy Book of Forensic Medicine and Toxicology," London, 1877, p. 623.

In many cases the teeth have constituted the most important part of the evidence by means of which the remains of a human being have been identified. Thus, the remains discovered among the ruins of Hatfield House after the fire were identified as being those of the Marchion-

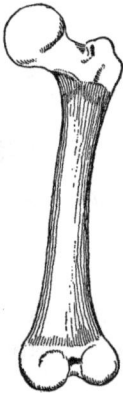

Fig. 7.—From a child at birth, showing a nucleus in the lower epiphysis.

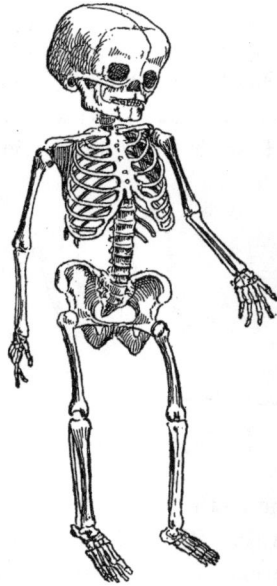

Fig. 8.—The skeleton of a child about one year old.

ess of Salisbury through the jaw-bone having gold appendages for artificial teeth. In another case that occurred in Edinburgh the identity of the deceased was established by the dentist, who produced a cast of the gums.* In the celebrated case of Dr. Parkman, who

* Guy and Ferrier: " Principles of Forensic Medicine," 1881, p. 26.

was murdered in Boston, the remains of the deceased were identified to a considerable extent by a set of artificial teeth made for Dr. Parkman three years before his death. Notwithstanding that an attempt had been made to burn the head, and that the gold had melted, the mineral teeth, being infusible, remained in such a good state of preservation that they were at once recognized by the dentist who made them.

The degree of ossification of the lower epiphysis of the femur (Fig. 7) is one of the most certain signs of the age of the fœtus and of the new-born child. * Thus, if no ossific deposit be found in the cartilaginous epiphysis of the femur, it may be stated that the fœtus has not yet reached the eighth month of intrauterine life. If the ossific deposit has attained a diameter of about one line, the fœtus has reached full term. If the ossific deposit measures more than one-quarter of an inch, the child has lived after birth for some little time. The length of the skeleton of the child at birth is usually about sixteen inches. Ossification begins at the extremities of most of the long bones at the end of the first year (Fig. 8), and progresses from that time on until ossification is completed. The epiphyses of all the long bones are usually found united to their shafts in the male at about twenty-four years, in the female at about twenty-two years.

After ossification has once been completed it is difficult, if possible, to determine exactly the age from an examination of the skeleton alone. It may be mentioned, however, that the bones of the sternum (Fig. 9)

* Béclard: "Nouvelle Journal de Médecine, Chirurgie, et Pharmacie," tome iv, 1819, p. 113; Casper: *op. cit.*, vol. iii, p. 23.

are usually found ununited until after forty,* those of the sacrum (Fig. 10) and os coccygis until sixty years of age. The height of a body may be approximately estimated from the skeleton, the latter being entire, by placing the bones in position and adding from one inch and a half to two inches to the length to supply the

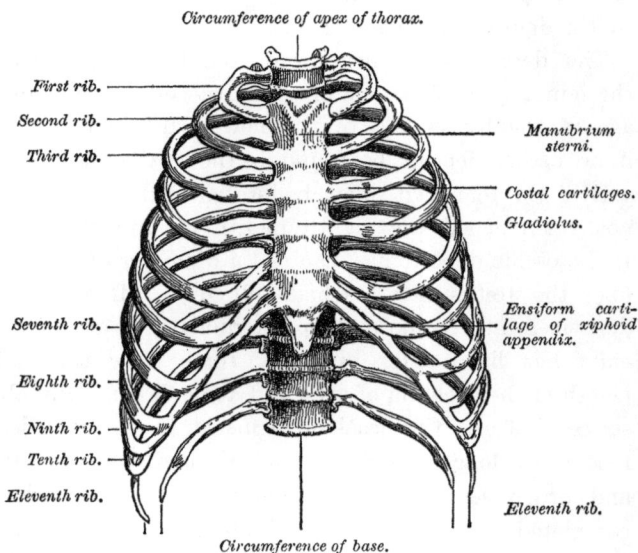

Circumference of apex of thorax.

First rib.
Second rib.
Third rib.

Manubrium sterni.

Costal cartilages.
Gladiolus.

Seventh rib.

Ensiform cartilage of xiphoid appendix.

Eighth rib.
Ninth rib.
Tenth rib.
Eleventh rib.

Eleventh rib.

Circumference of base.
Fig. 9.—Thorax, anterior view.

missing soft parts. In the absence of the skull there should be added about ten inches to the height of the spine of the seventh cervical vertebra from the ground.

A skeleton may be identified as that of some particular person even years after death, through the pres-

* Guy and Ferrier: *op. cit.*, London, 1881, p. 36; Wharton and Stillé: *op. cit.*, vol. ii:, p. 470.

ence of deformities, fractures, callus, etc. The production of callus is the result of the reparative process that takes place in the case of fractured bones, and its presence proves that some time must have elapsed between the time of fracture and death, a fact at times of great practical importance.

Thus, for example, in the case of a gentleman who was tried in India for the murder of a native, it was al-

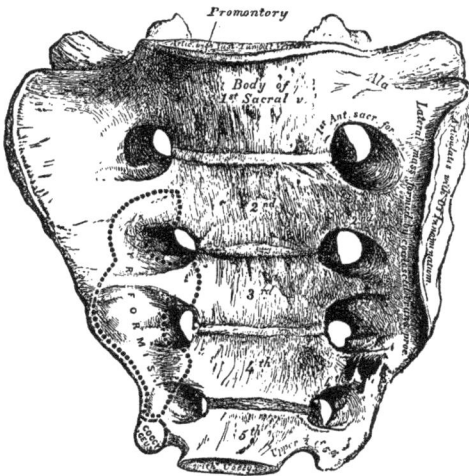

Fig. 10.—Sacrum, anterior surface (after Gray).

leged that the deceased had been struck several blows before his death, thereby breaking his ribs. On examination, however, of the skeleton said to be that of the deceased, it was found that while a rib had been fractured, it was united by a firm osseous callus, which proved very conclusively that the fracture of the rib could not have been due to the blow struck a few hours before death, but must have been caused in some other way some time previously. On the other hand, the absence of such callus in cases of death following fractures would clearly indicate that death followed soon after the injury causing the fracture. Under certain circumstances it may become a matter of importance to determine from an examination of the skeleton alone the length of time that the body has been buried. It may be said that, while ordinarily within ten years after burial the soft parts of a body entirely disappear, the bones, however, may resist decomposition for thirty or forty years, particularly if the surrounding soil is dry. It is well known, however, that the skeletons of individuals buried in leaden or in stone coffins have been found in a tolerable state of preservation even after a lapse of more than a thousand years. The bones of King Dagobert, for example, were disinterred from the Church of St. Denis after twelve hundred, skeletons from Pompeii after eighteen hundred years.*

The Coroner's Inquest and the Grand Jury.—After the coroner has held his inquest, and the coroner's physician and the witnesses have given their testimony, and the jury submitted their verdict, the defendant, in case of the verdict being "guilty," is then remanded to the district attorney's office. The case then comes up before the grand jury, to which the coroner's physician states substantially what he has already said at the coroner's inquest. If the grand jury finds a true bill, the case then goes to court, the trial is set for a certain day, and the coroner's physician is subpœnaed for the third time to appear in court.

* Guy and Ferrier: *op. cit.*, p. 29.

Conduct of Medical Witnesses in Court.—If the court is aware that the coroner's physician or any of the medical experts engaged in the case have large practice or are connected as lecturers with any particular medical schools, etc., it is very considerate, as a general rule, arranging its business so as to inconvenience them as little as possible. It is incumbent, however, upon the physician, whether he be the coroner's physician or retained as an expert for the defense, to treat the court with every possible respect, to be always punctual in attendance, and if he be unavoidably delayed by professional exigencies, to send the court word explaining the cause of non-attendance. The court, however, will not submit to any of the physicians subpœnaed straggling in at any hour of the day with no excuse to offer for their non-attendance but detention by their everyday practice.

At the trial, the medical witness, if he be the coroner's physician, is examined first by the prosecution, by the district attorney. Having given testimony, he is cross-examined by the counsel for the defense, and is then usually re-examined by the district attorney, and here, as a rule, his examination ends. In giving evidence in court a medical witness should always maintain a dignified, composed demeanor. He should never be arrogant or show any irritability, still less lose his temper, however much he may be annoyed by the examination or cross-examination. He should never forget that the object of the prosecution is to elicit all the evidence that will lead to conviction; the object of the defense to try to rebut, break down all that the prosecution hoped to establish. The medical witness should so answer that he can be heard by the whole court, addressing himself more particularly to the jury. His answers should be brief and given in the simplest language, all technical terms being avoided as much as possible. It is better for the medical examiner to say, for example, that he found on the brain a blood-clot rather than an apoplectic extravasation; a bruise, rather than a contusion, or an ecchymosis; to simply say that he removed the skin from the chest, rather than that he reflected the integument from the thorax and laid bare the costal cartilages. The medical examiner who observes that he found "a severe contusion of the integument under the left orbit, with great extravasation of blood and ecchymosis in the surrounding cellular tissue, which was in a tumefied state," etc., renders himself liable to be asked by the judge if he means by all that a black eye, and if so, why does he not say so.*

The medical witness who indulges in that kind of pedantry will soon learn that the court is not in the least impressed by it, and that good, plain English is far more appreciated. Finally, the witness should never be ashamed of saying in open court that he does not know. The court does not expect the witness to know everything. Nothing is more foolish for a witness than to hazard a guess in answer to a question for fear of being thought ignorant.

Dying declarations, it may be mentioned in this connection, are accepted in law as evidence without being sworn to. It is naturally presumed that all statements made at such a solemn crisis must be sincere, believed at least to be true by the dying person even if subsequently

* Taylor: *op. cit.,* p. 52.

shown not to be so. The attending physician under such circumstances having expressed the opinion that the patient is dying and in sound mind, a magistrate should be summoned to take down any statements that the dying person may wish to make. Should it not be possible to obtain the services of a magistrate, then the attending physician can take down the dying declarations. The physician should, however, limit himself to writing down the exact words of the dying person without offering any interpretation whatever. The statement should be read over to the dying person, and, if possible, his signature to it obtained.

Wills.—In cases where the attending physician is called upon in an emergency to draft or witness a will for a patient, it is essential that he clearly understand the wishes of the testator, that he ascertain the bodily and mental condition of the latter, secure the testator's signature and affix his own as a witness, and note all the circumstances bearing upon the case, so that in the event of the will being disputed he can testify intelligently and stand a searching cross-examination when the case is tried.

CHAPTER IV.

Medico-legal Definition of Wounds—Comparison of Wounds with Weapons Inflicting Them and Clothes of Deceased—Incised, Contused, Penetrating Wounds—Suicidal, Homicidal, Accidental Wounds—Gunshot Wounds—Causes of Death from Wounds.

Medico-legal Definition of Wounds.—A wound, from a purely surgical point of view, is regarded as a solution of continuity of the soft parts occasioned by external violence. The medico-legal idea of a wound is, however, far more comprehensive, embracing all injuries of the body, external or internal, with or without a solution of continuity of the skin, produced suddenly by external violence.* As the danger of a wound will depend on the age and constitution of the person, its position, the weapon by which it was inflicted, the amount of hemorrhage, and numerous other circumstances, it is impossible for a physician to state positively whether a wound will prove fatal or not. Wounds at first apparently trivial have subsequently, in many cases, as is well known, been the cause of death. The medical witness should, therefore, express himself most cautiously if he replies at all to the questions so often asked, "Will such a wound prove fatal?" "Was such a wound necessarily mortal?"

In making a post-mortem examination in cases where death is due to wounds, it is most important that the

* Beck, T. B. and J. B.: *op. cit.*, vol. ii, p. 282.

medical examiner should satisfy himself, not only that the wound was the cause of death, but also that the remaining organs were healthy, or at least were not in such a condition that death could be attributed in any way to them; indeed, or to any cause other than the one assigned. On more than one occasion has the defendant been acquitted owing to such neglect giving rise in the minds of the jury to the doubt as to whether disease or the wound was the real cause of death. On the other hand, a defendant may run the risk of being convicted of murder if it was in evidence that violence had been offered to the deceased, the true cause of death, disease, not having been shown, owing to the superficial character of the post-mortem examination.

The importance of making a thorough post-mortem examination in cases of death from violence is well shown in cases of persons crushed to death, as by a heavily loaded wagon. It is well known that, although the external signs of violence in such cases may be limited to a few abrasions, the internal injuries causing death may be of the most extensive and serious character. Thus, in the well-known case described by Casper, of the man who was crushed to death between his wagon, heavily laden with glass, and a poplar tree, nothing was observed externally but a trifling abrasion of the cuticle over the right cheek-bone and a similar one upon the left arm; yet upon opening the thorax thirty ounces of dark fluid blood escaped, the heart was found torn from the great blood-vessels lying loose at the bottom of the thoracic cavity, the pericardium having been completely torn across the left lung, almost divided in the middle, and a laceration of the right lobe of the liver two inches long and half an inch deep. Further, the spinous process of the first thoracic vertebra was found broken and lying loose in the soft parts, while about a quart of dark fluid blood escaped from the spinal canal.*

Comparison of Wounds with Weapons.—In deaths from wounds the medical examiner should note their exact situation, direction, and extent. If the weapon by which the wounds were known or supposed to have been inflicted has been obtained, it should be compared with the wounds themselves, so that, on subsequent examination, he can positively state whether such wounds as were found might have been inflicted by the weapon submitted. We say "might" and not "were" inflicted, as the medical examiner should never say positively that a wound was inflicted by a particular weapon, even though the latter fitted the wound exactly, since it might be proved later that the wound had been caused by some other weapon. Thus, in a well-known case where a man stabbed another, the medical witness testified positively that the wound was caused by a knife with a perfectly entire blade that was submitted in evidence. Twelve months afterward an abscess, formed in the situation of the wound, opened, and discharged the point of a knife, proving conclusively that the wound had not been caused by the knife submitted in evidence.†

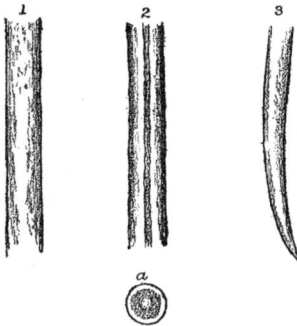

Fig. 11.—Human hair: 1, The hair of a child; 2, hair of an adult; 3, pointed extremity of the hair of the eyebrow; *a*, transverse section of the hair, showing the cortical and medullary portion, and air-cells in the center of the cylinder.

* Casper: *op. cit.*, vol. i, p. 112, case xl.
† Woodman and Tidy: *op. cit.*, p. 1090.

The clothes of the deceased should be carefully inspected, and any rents, cuts, or tears found, compared with the wounds in the body, and with the weapon by which they were said to be inflicted, as such an examination may throw light upon the cause of death. Thus, for example, a woman was found dead in her bed who had been seen apparently well the previous night, with two indentations in the parietal region of the head and blood on the floor, which had flowed from the nose. On post-mortem examination death was found to be due to a fracture of the parietal bone. It was in evidence that the woman was accidentally knocked down the evening before her death, she falling heavily on the back of her head, upon which at the time she wore a bonnet. At first she was stunned, but soon recovered, and after taking some brandy walked home and ate her supper as usual, after which she was not seen again until found dead the following morning. From the fact that the deceased and a fellow-lodger had been in the habit of quarreling and that the latter had in his possession a hammer with two claws, which the medical examiner testified could have produced the two indentations and the fracture of the parietal bone, the fellow-lodger was suspected of having murdered the woman, he being the only other person in the house at that time. At the adjourned inquest, however, the bonnet worn by the deceased at the time of the accident was put in evidence by the coroner, and it was then shown that it presented two indentations filled with dust and dirt, which corresponded with the two indentations in the head of the deceased, thereby confirming the statements of the witnesses and rendering it highly probable that death was due to the fall. This case illustrates well the caution that the medical examiner should

5

exercise in testifying as to the manner in which wounds are produced, and also that a person may walk a considerable distance and live some time after receiving a serious injury of the head.*

Hairs, fibers, etc., found upon the weapon supposed to have inflicted the fatal wound, or upon the person of the accused, should be examined with the microscope and compared with those of the clothing worn by the deceased, as such examination may lead to the conviction of the accused, as was the case in the following instance: A girl nine years

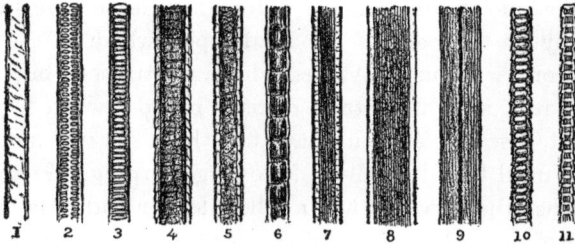

Fig. 12.—Microscopic appearance of hairs of various animals: 1, Hair of the spaniel; 2, hair or fur of the rabbit; 3, hair of the hare; 4, hair of the horse; 5, hair of the goat; 6, hair of the fox; 7, hair of the cow; 8, hair of the fallow deer; 9, hair of the ox; 10, hair of the cat; 11, hair of the mouse.

old was found dead at Norwich, England, with her throat cut. Her mother, being suspected of having murdered the child, was arrested, but coolly explained the absence of the child by supposing that she had lost her way picking flowers. Upon being searched, however, a long, sharp knife was found in the possession of the woman, to which adhered a few pieces of hair, the presence of which the woman explained by saying that the hairs were those of a rabbit that she had killed on her way home. On examina-

* Wharton and Stillé: *op. cit.*, vol. ii, p. 271.

tion with the microscope, however, these hairs were shown to be those of a squirrel, and it was in evidence that the child wore at the time of her death, around her neck, a tippet made of squirrel fur, through which the knife, by whomever held, must have passed at the time that the child's throat was cut.

Further, blood was found between the horn handle of the knife and its iron lining, that was held by the microscopist to resemble human blood. On this evidence the mother was convicted and before execution confessed that she had murdered her child.*

As a general rule, human hairs (Fig. 11) can readily be distinguished from those of animals, or from fibers of cotton, silk, wool, etc. The hairs of the lower animals, some of which

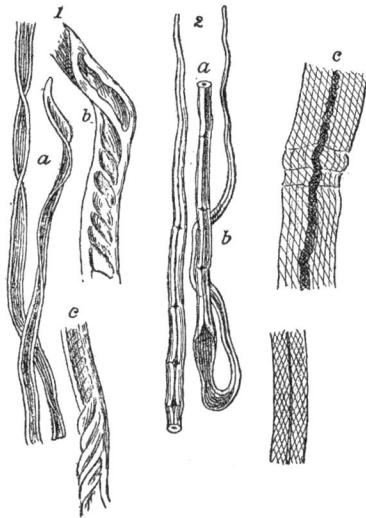

Fig. 13.—1. Cotton: a, normal condition; b, portion treated with sulphuric acid and iodin; c, fragment of guncotton. 2. Flax: a, normal fiber; b, portion boiled with nitric acid; c, treated with nitric acid and afterward with sulphuric acid and iodin.

are represented in figure 12, differ in many respects from those of man, being generally coarser, thicker, shorter, and less transparent. Microscopically, the most striking differences in hairs are presented by the cells and linear markings of their cortical portions. The fibers of cotton (Fig. 13, 1)

* Taylor: *op. cit.*, p. 261.

are flattened bands disposed in a spiral or twisted manner. Those of flax (Fig. 13, 2) are rectilinear, tapering to a point and presenting pointed markings at unequal distances. Silk fibers are cylindrical in shape, almost entirely free from markings, and refract light powerfully. The fibers of wool are rather irregular in form and unequal in thickness.

Character of Wounds.—Wounds are usually described as being incised, lacerated, contused, punctured, or penetrating. Incised wounds may generally be recognized by the regularity and evenness of the cut; and it might naturally be supposed that they would be made by cutting weapons, contused wounds by blunt ones, and penetrating wounds by pointed instruments. It must be admitted that in certain cases, as in wounds inflicted by broken glass or china, which often resemble exactly incised wounds, it might be very difficult to say how the wounds had been made. Indeed, it is impossible for the medical examiner, though often asked, to state positively whether a wound was or was not inflicted with a particular kind of weapon.

Wounds before or after Death.—It often becomes important to determine whether a wound was inflicted before or after death. In the case of an incised wound this is usually not very difficult, since, if made before death, the edges of the wound will be found everted and the latter more or less filled with coagulated blood, principally of an arterial character, or with granulations, pus, or sloughs, if any length of time has elapsed before death. Too much importance should not be attached to the presence of coagulated blood as a proof of a wound having been inflicted during life, since, as is well known, blood drawn from the dead will coagulate as well as that from the living body.*

In those cases in which death is practically instantaneous, life becoming extinct before any reparative material is produced, it becomes not only difficult, but often impossible to distinguish such wounds from those made after death. Thus, in the case often cited of a woman who was killed almost instantly by the thrusting of a table knife between the first and second ribs through the arch of the aorta, the wound presented smooth and sharp edges without a trace of fluid or dried blood, resembling in every respect a wound made upon the dead body.†

Contused wounds, if made during life, are characterized by ecchymoses, suggillation, or the black-and-blue discoloration due to the rupture of the small vessels, and the effusion of blood into the cellular tissue under the skin. The progressive changes of color—purple, black, violet, green, yellow—exhibited by ecchymoses serve not only to indicate whether the bruise was made before or after death, but also as to the length of time elapsing since its production. Thus, for example, within twelve hours after the injury, and in some cases immediately afterward, the color presented by the bruise is that of a purplish-black; by the third day it has become violet; by the fifth or sixth day, green; and by from the eighth to the tenth day, yellow. The latter color gradually disappears by from the twelfth to the fourteenth day, the skin reassuming its natural hue and presenting no trace of its discoloration.

It should be mentioned that blows inflicted within two hours after death may give rise to discoloration of the

* Casper: *op. cit.*, vol. I, p. 24.
† Casper: *op. cit.*, vol. I, p. 121.

skin resembling so closely those produced during life, except in being less in extent, as to deceive even expert examiners in regard to their true origin. Indeed, the discolorations of the skin produced by Christison by blows made upon the body of a dead woman were so like those made by blows inflicted usually during life that the attendants of the dead-house who received the body of the deceased refused to allow it to be buried, so convinced were they that the woman had been beaten to death. Further, in some cases ecchymosis may not appear at all until after death. Thus, for example, in the case of a person who died with rupture of the bladder thirty-five hours after being kicked by a horse, there was no discoloration of the skin until after death. The medical examiner should be cautious, therefore, in stating positively whether a bruise was produced by a blow inflicted before or after death.

The situation, extent, and direction of a wound and the position in which the weapon was found, in regard to the body of the deceased, should be most carefully observed and noted, as they may lead to the determining of whether the wound was suicidal, homicidal, or accidental.

Suicidal Wounds.—In cases of persons taking their own lives, the mouth, forehead, the region over the heart, etc., are usually chosen if firearms are used; the throat or heart if the wounds are inflicted with cutting instruments. While ordinarily accessible parts of the body are selected by suicides, it must not be forgotten that insane persons, in committing suicide, have inflicted wounds upon themselves in most inaccessible parts, such as the back of the head and neck. It is well known that insane persons have killed themselves by falling backward, their heads striking upon some hard substances, or by fracturing the posterior part of their skull with a cleaver or hatchet. Such cases would naturally suggest the idea of murder having been committed had the bodies been found in some deserted place and were it not in evidence that death was due to suicide. Insane persons not infrequently also shoot themselves through the back of the head, a fact that should not be lost sight of, in that such a wound would naturally suggest that it was a homicide. Incised wounds of the throat, especially if the direction of the wound be from left to right, the deceased being right-handed, are usually regarded as presumptive of the death being suicidal.

Homicidal Wounds.—It should be remembered that a very common way of committing murder is by cutting the throat of the victim, the murderer standing behind; a wound inflicted in such a manner would resemble that committed by a suicide. On the other hand, the irregularity of the wound often observed in such cases, and sometimes submitted as a proof that the wound was homicidal, and attributable to the resistance offered by the deceased in his struggle for life, might just as well be accounted for on the supposition that it was suicidal and due to the nervousness and indecision of the deceased. A homicidal can often be distinguished from a suicidal wound by its direction. Thus, for example, a man was found dead with a wound in the neck, of such a character that it was positively stated by the medical examiner that the weapon had been partially turned and withdrawn, and again plunged into the neck in a different direction, according to the manner of German butchers, which evidence not only proved that the wound was not due to suicide or accident, but to murder, and also indicated the occupation of the murderer.*   As another

* Kopp's "Jahrbücher," erster Jahrgang, 1808, S. 143.

illustration of the importance of determining exactly the direction of a wound, it may be mentioned that some years ago a butcher was convicted of murder in England, it being shown by the medical examiner that the wound had been made from within to without, as is done by English butchers in the killing of sheep.*

Accidental wounds are apt to occur among crowds in fighting, when the deceased is thrown or falls against some hard, resisting body. Death may be attributed plausibly to accident in cases when the bodies of the deceased are found near precipices, in ravines, in rivers with steep banks, especially when it is known that the deceased had been addicted to the abuse of alcohol.

Wounds produced accidentally are usually found in such parts of the body as are exposed. Bruises, fractures, or dislocations would suggest, therefore, that death was due to accident rather than to incised, punctured, or lacerated wounds, though not necessarily so. If wounds the nature of which might otherwise lead to the supposition that they had been made accidentally are found upon both sides of the body, the presumption would then be that they were homicidal.

Gunshot wounds are essentially contusions. Owing to the vitality of the parts struck being destroyed by the projectile, there ensues a process of sloughing. In this respect gunshot wounds differ from ordinary wounds. They differ very much in appearance, according to the nature of the projectile, to the distance from which the piece was discharged, etc. As a general rule the hemorrhage following a gunshot wound is not very great, unless some of the large vessels are wounded. It should be mentioned

* Wharton and Stillé: *op. cit.*, vol. III, p. 241.

that though the external hemorrhage may not be very great, owing to the form and size of the wound, the internal hemorrhage may be so severe as to prove fatal. If the weapon be in immediate contact with the body at the moment that it was discharged, the wound made is large, the skin is denuded, blackened, and partly burned. The hair or the clothes are also usually scorched. The aperture of entrance of the missile, if it be a ball, is depressed and larger than that of the exit orifice.

It must be admitted that considerable difference of opinion still prevails among medical jurists as to whether the entrance aperture of the ball is larger or smaller than the exit one. This may be due possibly to the relative distance of the weapon and the body not being taken sufficiently into consideration, the entrance aperture being said to be larger than the exit one when the weapon is close to the body, but smaller when the weapon is at some distance —twelve paces or so—from it.* It should be stated, that according to some authorities the exit aperture is invariably larger than the entrance one whatever the distance of the weapon from the body.† It must be borne in mind, also, that the entrance aperture may appear to be smaller than that of the bullet making it, owing to the elasticity of the living skin; and the same is true of an opening made in clothing composed of elastic material.

The character of the entrance aperture of the wound will depend upon the shape of the missile, the velocity with which it was traveling, and the distance from which it was fired. Thus, a wound made by a conoidal ball, like that of a

---

* Wharton and Stillé: *op. cit.*, vol. III, p. 233.

† Casper: *op. cit.*, vol. I, p. 266; Woodman and Tidy: *op. cit.*, p. 1115.

Minié rifle, is linear in form. Such a wound produces but little external, though considerable internal, injury. On the other hand, the wound made by a rifle ball is ragged and large. A ball, after entering the body, may, as is well known, be so deflected from its course by striking a bone or a tendon, etc., as to pass entirely around the body and so reach finally the point of entrance. If a gunshot wound be caused by a load of shot, the appearance presented will depend upon the distance from which the shot was fired. If the weapon discharged be within twelve inches of the body, the wound will usually be a single one. Beyond that distance each shot will make a single individual wound,* and one or two grains of shot may even cause death. Thus, a thief, while endeavoring to escape by climbing a wall, received a charge of shot from a fowling-piece at a distance of fifteen paces and fell dead. The charge, having entered the chest, scattered over an extent of three to four inches, one grain of shot penetrating the aorta at the level of the semilunar valves, the others traversing the anterior wall of the vessel.†

Serious, if not fatal, wounds may be caused by wadding and gunpowder alone if the weapon be within three or four inches of the body.

Causes of Death from Wounds.—With reference to the committing of suicide by means of firearms, it may be mentioned that in four-fifths of the cases the part of the body selected for the infliction of the wounds is the head, the mouth being the part more particularly chosen. Thus, out of 368 cases of suicide by firearms reported by De Bois-

* Lachese: "Annales de Hygiene publique," Paris, 1836, p 359; Casper: *op. cit.*, vol. I, p. 266.

† Wharton and Stillé: *op. cit.*, vol. III, p. 237.

mont,* in 297 cases the head was the part wounded, in 71 cases only the chest or the abdomen. Of the first group, in 234 cases the weapon was fired into the mouth.

Under certain circumstances it may become important for the medical examiner to be able to state, in the case of death from wounds, the remote as well as the immediate cause of death. The immediate cause of death from a wound is either hemorrhage or shock, the latter being the result of a powerful impression made upon the nervous centers. Of the remote causes of death from wounds the most common are tetanus or lockjaw, erysipelas, hospital gangrene, surgical operations, including the use of ether or chloroform. The danger of wounds depends, to a great extent, upon the parts of the body affected. Thus, scalp wounds are not usually dangerous unless followed by erysipelas. It should be remembered, however, in cases of wounds of the head, that a fracture or effusion of blood upon the brain, or concussion, may be produced by a blow, even though the scalp be uninjured. It is most important that the effects of concussion should not be mistaken for those of intoxication. Unfortunately, in too many instances persons arrested upon the charge of intoxication have died in station-houses from concussion of the brain, when their lives might have been saved had medical attendance been summoned.

Wounds of the face are not usually dangerous unless the orbit be involved. In a case in which the post-mortem examination was made by the author, death was shown to have been caused by inflammation of the brain due to the penetration of the orbital plate by the point of an um-

* De Boismont: "Du Suicide," deuxième edition, Paris, 1865, p. 681.

brella thrust into the face. The danger of wounds of the neck is due to the presence of the great vessels, the division of which, in the case of the throat, gives rise to severe hemorrhage. The trachea and larynx may be divided, however, without necessarily proving fatal, unless the blood flows into the trachea in such quantity as to cause death. Death

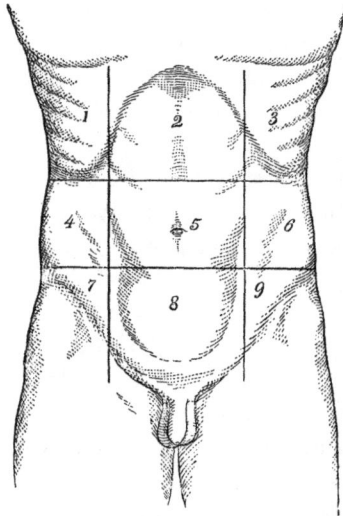

Fig. 14.—Imaginary lines drawn upon the surface of the abdomen dividing it into regions. *1*, Right hypochondriac region ; *2*, epigastric ; *3*, left hypochondriac ; *4*, right lumbar; *5*, umbilical; *6*, left lumbar; *7*, right iliac; *8*, hypogastric; *9*, left iliac.

from wounds of the chest is usually due to hemorrhage from the heart, lungs, or great vessels. In cases of wounds of the abdomen, involving the liver, stomach, or intestines (see Fig. 14, regions 1, 2, 3), the cause of death is frequently peritonitis.

With regard to wounds of the bladder (see Fig. 14, region

8) it must be borne in mind that, if distended, it may readily be ruptured by a blow upon the abdomen, the cause of death being usually peritonitis. Frequently, however, under such circumstances there may be no signs of external injury. In wounds of the spine the danger is proportional to the extent to which the spinal cord is involved, death taking place instantaneously if the medulla or upper portion of the spinal cord is wounded. The danger in wounds of the generative organs is due to the severe hemorrhage which usually ensues. In the male sex, in the case of the insane, castration and amputation of the penis are frequently self-inflicted.

CHAPTER V.

Blood-stains—Chemical, Microscopic, and Spectroscopic Methods of Investigation—Coagulation of Blood—Conditions Influencing Coagulation—Amount of Blood in the Body.

NOT infrequently, in cases of murder, it becomes necessary to determine whether certain dark stains, such as are found on a knife, linen, underwear, pieces of wood, etc., were made by blood. The appearance presented by blood-stains will vary according to their size, shape, and color. Usually the stain consists of distinct spots; it may, however, be a mere streak or film. The color of recent blood-stains is red, due to the hæmoglobin effused from the red corpuscles; that of old ones, brown or brownish-red, the hæmoglobin having been converted into methæmoglobin or hæmatin. It must be mentioned, however, that the fact of a blood-stain being brown does not necessarily prove that it is old, since there are other conditions not well understood that modify the color of blood-stains as well as age. A blood-stain will be more or less modified according to the nature of the material upon which the blood has fallen. Thus, the color of blood upon soft wool, linen, or cloth is dark; that upon a polished metallic surface is shining, the spots presenting in the latter case cracks radiating from the center.

Methods of Examining Blood-stains.—There are three methods of examining stains supposed to have been made by blood—the chemical, the microscopic, and the spectroscopic—all of which, on account of the importance of the subject, demand description.

The *chemical method* of investigation is based upon the fact that the hæmoglobin of the red corpuscles of the blood is soluble in cold water. If the suspected blood-stain is in sufficient quantity and not so old that the hæmoglobin has been converted into hæmatin, which is insoluble, by proper manipulation a solution of the coloring-matter of the blood can be obtained and then tested. If the article stained be a linen shirt, for example, a small piece should be cut out and suspended in a test-tube containing cold distilled water. In a few minutes, or longer, if the stain be an old one, the coloring-matter of the blood will pass into the water, coloring it red. If the stained material to be examined is attached to wood or a knife-blade, it must be scraped or cut off and then soaked in water. Should the solution be incomplete, a trace of citric acid or a little ammonia may be added, the latter not affecting the color of the solution. The solution so obtained should then be heated in a test-tube over a spirit-lamp. If the solution be that of the coloring-matter of the blood, it will coagulate, the red color will disappear, and a brownish-green material will be precipitated. By adding liquor potassæ the clot will be dissolved and a solution will be obtained that appears dark green by transmitted and red by reflected light, the clot reappearing on the addition of nitric acid. In this way a solution of the coloring-matter of the blood may usually be distinguished from other red solutions, such as those of red prints, logwood, kino, madder, cochineal, colored infusions of flowers and roots, and the juices of fruits, which do not coagulate when heated, and which change their color when ammonia is added.

Stains made by red paint or by lemon-juice on iron, while slightly resembling blood-stains, can be distinguished from the latter through their color becoming a bluish, inky black on addition of tincture of galls, ferrocyanide of potassium, or by other tests for iron. This is a fact of some practical importance, as illustrated by the case of a man who was suspected of murder on account of a knife, apparently covered with blood, being found in his possession. On examination, however, the stains were shown to be due to citric acid, the knife having been used a few days before to cut a lemon and having been put away unwiped. •

An important test for blood among the chemical tests, on account of it being reliable and readily performed, is that known as the guaiacum test, based upon the fact that the resin of guaiacum when oxidized assumes a sapphire-blue color, and that this change in the color of the resin can be induced by the addition of blood and peroxide of hydrogen together, but not by the addition of blood alone. A convenient way of applying the guaiacum test, frequently made use of by the writer, is to add a few drops of a freshly prepared tincture of guaiacum to a small quantity of water, by which the resin is precipitated. The water holding the resin in suspension is then divided into three portions. To the first portion a few drops of peroxide of hydrogen dissolved in ether are added; to the second portion, a few drops of the solution supposed to contain the coloring-matter of the blood. In neither case will any change in the color of the resin be observed. Now to the third portion add a few drops of the suspected solution and of the etherized peroxide and at once the resin will assume a sapphire-blue color. Should the solution be turbid through excess of the resin, a few drops of alcohol will instantly clear it. It should be mentioned in this connection that the resin of guaiacum in the presence of peroxid of hydrogen is oxidized, turns blue by the addition of bile, saliva, red wine, as well as by blood. The color of bile and saliva, however, should serve to distinguish these secretions from blood, while in the case of red wine several hours are required to produce the blue color in the resin. It will be observed that the existence of blood is not directly proved by the chemical tests just described, but is inferred from the presence of its coloring-matter or hæmoglobin, and in most cases is only presumptively established.

In recent years it has been shown that rabbits having been previously injected subcutaneously with human blood or blood-serum will yield a serum which will give a " precepitum " with human blood, but not with the blood of the rabbit, guinea-pig, horse, sheep, or ox, and the hope has been expressed that this test may serve in the future as a delicate means of detecting blood in medico-legal cases.* It is very doubtful, however, whether the presence of blood could be satisfactorily established by the "precepitum" test with the kind of material suspected to be blood that is usually submitted to the medical expert; and even in the event of that test proving the presence of blood, it would not prove necessarily that it was human blood, since the blood of several species of monkeys responds to the test as well as that of man.

The *microscopic method* of proving the existence of blood depends on the ability of the examiner to treat the material submitted to him, which does not consist of freshly drawn

* V. C. Vaughan and F. G. Novy: "Cellular Toxins," fourth edition, 1902, pp. 119–121.

6

blood, but of material supposed to have been stained with blood, in such a way that if it be blood the corpuscles, and more especially the red ones, may be sufficiently restored to admit of identification under the microscope, or at least to enable him to obtain the crystalline forms developed through changes in their coloring-matter. The separation of the corpuscles from a material consisting of pieces of linen, wood, or iron stained with blood mixed with dirt, etc., is a far more difficult operation, however, than that of demonstrating simply the presence of blood-crystals. If the material submitted for examination is a piece of linen, for example, stained with what is supposed to be blood, a piece of it should be cut out and placed upon a clean glass slide and moistened with a solution consisting of one part of glycerin to seven of water, or with a solution of common salt having a specific gravity of that of the serum of the blood—1.055–1.063. The specimen should then be covered with a thin cover-glass and examined with the microscope. By this method, if the stain be blood, and not too old, the red blood-corpuscles, and sometimes the white ones as well, will be usually brought into view. If the material suspected to be blood is in the form of a clot, on a knife-blade, for example, a small portion of it should be scraped off with a needle on to a perfectly clean glass slide. A thin cover-glass being pressed firmly down on the fragment until it is reduced to powder, the glass slide is then placed upon the stage of the microscope. A drop of distilled water being allowed to flow slowly from the margin of the cover-glass toward the powdered material, if the latter be blood, the corpuscles will gradually make their appearance, and, although faint and colorless, are usually sufficiently definite in outline to admit of identification.

A red blood-corpuscle of man (Fig. 15), as seen in freshly drawn blood, may be described as a biconcave disk, a mass or cell of protoplasm without a cell-wall or nucleus, and with a diameter in its greatest width on an average of $\frac{1}{3200}$ of an inch.

Micrometer.—Inasmuch as there are obtained from supposed blood-stains certain bodies having the size just mentioned, and as this is usually regarded as one of the strongest proofs that such bodies are red blood-corpuscles, the method by which they are measured must be described. The instrument used for this purpose by the microscopist is an eyepiece micrometer—that is, an eyepiece upon the glass of which have been ruled a number of parallel and equidistant lines, which, on being projected upon the field of the microscope, will be seen by the observer to cover any objects visible there and to define their limits. To use the eyepiece micrometer the value of the spaces between the lines

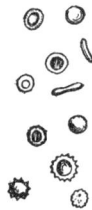

Fig. 15.—Blood-corpuscles ($\times$ 450).

must be determined for the particular magnification, since these will vary with the objective and the length of tube used. To accomplish this there is placed upon the stage of the microscope a glass slide upon which have been ruled a number of parallel lines separated from one another by distances of $\frac{1}{10}$, $\frac{1}{100}$, and $\frac{1}{1000}$ of an inch respectively (Fig. 16). Let us suppose, for example, that the magnifying power used is such that ten lines of the eyepiece micrometer correspond exactly to the space between two of the lines upon the stage micrometer that are separated by $\frac{1}{1000}$ of an inch; the value of the spaces between the lines of the eyepiece micrometer will then be equal to $\frac{1}{10000}$ of an inch, and an object covered by four such spaces, as a white corpuscle (Fig. 16, W), would have a diameter, therefore, of $\frac{4}{10000} = \frac{1}{2500}$ of an inch. It is obvious, however, that with such magnification a red blood-corpuscle, if its diameter be $\frac{1}{3200}$ of an inch, will be covered by less than four such spaces, and by more than three, since $\frac{1}{3200}$ of an inch is less than $\frac{4}{10000}$ and more than $\frac{3}{10000}$ of an inch. As the red corpuscles, in order to be measured, must lie within the space between two lines the value of which is known, and further, as the edges of the corpuscle must be exactly in contact with the two lines circumscribing it, an object-glass

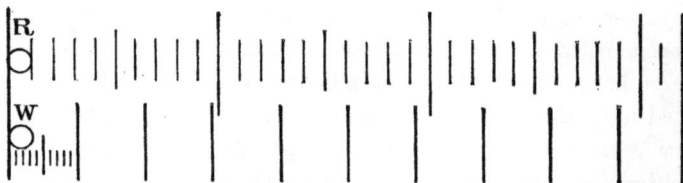

Fig. 16.—Lines of eyepiece micrometer, projected upon stage micrometer, as seen with different magnification.

and length of tube must be used so that exactly thirty-two lines of the eyepiece micrometer can be counted within a space of $\frac{1}{100}$ of an inch, as each space will then be equal to $\frac{1}{3200}$ of an inch, and will exactly cover the red corpuscles (Fig. 16, R).

A simple micrometric arrangement as that just described (Fig. 16) will suffice for determining whether bodies supposed to be red corpuscles have an average diameter of $\frac{1}{3200}$ of an inch, and, approximately at least, the diameter of larger or smaller bodies. It is obvious, however, that if the body to be measured was $\frac{1}{3000}$ of an inch in diameter, in order to measure it accurately the magnification (Fig. 16) would have to be so altered that the space of $\frac{1}{100}$ of an inch would contain exactly thirty lines instead of thirty-two. To avoid the inconvenience of altering the magnification in each case—which alteration would necessitate altering the length of the tube or changing the objective, or both—microscopists make use of a form of micrometer essentially the same as that used by astronomers in measuring the apparent diameters of the heavenly bodies. This consists of an ocular (Fig. 17, 1) through which may be seen projected upon the stage micrometer a fixed line A, and a movable line b. The latter can be moved across the field of the microscope by means of a wheel (not represented in the figure), the distance traversed by the thread b from the fixed line being determined by the number of divisions through which the wheel is rotated (Fig. 17, 3). As an illustration of the manner in which this is accomplished, let us suppose that the thread b is made to coincide with the fixed line A of the ocular, and the latter is made to coincide at the same time with the line B of the stage micrometer (Fig. 17, 2), and that the wheel is turned through one hundred divisions; that is, makes one complete rotation. It will be observed that the line b will traverse the space between the lines B and C of the stage micrometer, stopping at and coinciding with the line C. By the turning of the wheel through one hundred ·divisions the line b has, therefore, been made to traverse the space of $\frac{1}{100}$ of an inch, the space between B and C of the stage micrometer having been so graduated; consequently, if the wheel be turned through ten divisions, the limb b will be made to traverse $\frac{1}{1000}$ of an inch, and so on proportionally. The relation between the space traversed by the line b of the ocular and the number of divisions through which the wheel is turned having been experimentally determined by means of the stage micrometer, the latter is removed, and the object-glass holding

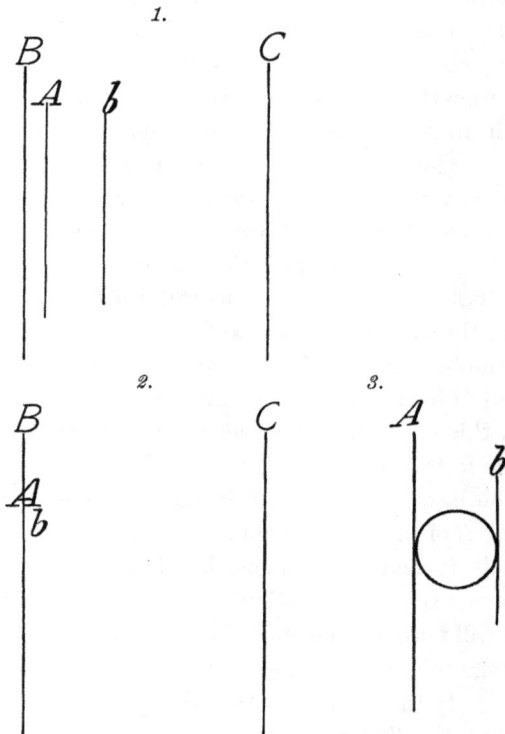

Fig. 17.—*B, C,* Lines upon stage micrometer; *A,* fixed line in ocular; *b,* movable line in ocular.

the object to be measured is substituted in the field of the microscope. To determine the size of the latter, it is only necessary then to turn the wheel until the body to be measured (Fig. 17, 3) is exactly circumscribed by the fixed line

A and the movable line b of the ocular, and to read off the number of divisions through which the wheel has been turned to accomplish this; for example, $\frac{1}{100}$ of an inch: 100 divisions of wheel : : x : 20 divisions:

$$x = \tfrac{1}{500} \text{ of an inch} = \text{diameter of body.}$$

It is evident, however, that if the wheel must be rotated through twenty divisions and a fraction of a division in order to bring the body to be measured between the lines A and b, that fraction might be such that even with a vernier attached to the wheel it would be impossible to get an exact reading, and consequently the measurement would only be approximate.

It is a matter, however, of the greatest difficulty with high powers to adjust accurately the divisions of the eye-piece micrometer, whatever form of instrument may be used, to either those of the stage micrometer or to the margins of the objects to be measured, even with all the ingenious accessory contrivances that have been devised to facilitate the operation.   Indeed, it must be admitted that the measurement of so small a body as the red corpuscle, even when made by a most skilful microscopist and with the best of modern instruments, from the very nature of the case is often only an approximate one.   If the measurement of the red blood-corpuscle from freshly drawn blood and under the most favorable circumstances is at best approximative, then how much more so must such measurement be in the case of a blood-stain where the size of the blood-corpuscle will depend upon the relative amount of the fluid absorbed that was used in separating it from the material that had previously contained it!

Admitting for the moment that the size of the body

supposed to be a blood-corpuscle has been correctly measured, how can the observer be sure that such diameter represents the diameter of the body in its original condition in a state of nature, since if the body had absorbed more of the fluid used in liberating it from the stain it would be larger, and if less, smaller? Indeed, one of the greatest difficulties experienced in restoring the form of the blood-corpuscles obtained from a blood-stain is to prevent their becoming distorted, swollen, or even bursting from excessive absorption of the fluid used in their preparation. On the other hand, if the body supposed to be the corpuscle does not absorb the normal amount of fluid, the observer measures the body before it reattains its full size.

The size of a corpuscle, as obtained from a blood-stain, can only be regarded, then, as representing approximately the size of the corpuscles of such blood. Further, it must be borne in mind, in this connection, that while about ninety out of every hundred red corpuscles, whether the blood be that of man or other mammals, have the same diameter, the latter depending upon the species, of the remaining ten corpuscles some are larger, some smaller than the average corpuscle. That being the case, if it just so happened that only the exceptionally small corpuscles were present, the blood, though human, might be erroneously regarded, on account of the small size of the corpuscles, as that of a dog, for example, in which the corpuscles are smaller than those of man. (See table.) On the other hand, if the blood examined was that of a dog, but only the exceptionally large corpuscles were obtained, such blood, on account of the large size of its corpuscles, might improperly be considered as human.

TABLE OF BLOOD-CORPUSCLES (DIAMETERS IN FRACTIONS OF AN INCH).

MAMMALS.

	DIAMETER.
Manatee	$\frac{1}{2700}$
Elephant	$\frac{1}{2745}$
Ant-eater	$\frac{1}{2769}$
Sloth	$\frac{1}{2865}$
Whale	$\frac{1}{3099}$
Camel	$\frac{1}{3123}$
Man	$\frac{1}{3200}$
Orang	$\frac{1}{3333}$
Chimpanzee	$\frac{1}{3412}$
Dog	$\frac{1}{3542}$
Opossum	$\frac{1}{3557}$
Rabbit	$\frac{1}{3607}$
Black rat	$\frac{1}{3754}$
Mouse	$\frac{1}{3814}$
Brown rat	$\frac{1}{3911}$
Gray squirrel	$\frac{1}{4000}$
Ox	$\frac{1}{4267}$
Cat	$\frac{1}{4404}$
Sheep	$\frac{1}{5300}$
Goat	$\frac{1}{6366}$
Pigmy musk deer	$\frac{1}{12325}$

BIRDS.

	DIAMETER.
Ostrich	$\frac{1}{1649}$
Owl	$\frac{1}{1763}$
Swan	$\frac{1}{1806}$
Pigeon	$\frac{1}{1973}$

REPTILES.

Turtle	$\frac{1}{1231}$
Viper	$\frac{1}{1274}$
Lizard	$\frac{1}{1555}$

AMPHIBIA.

Amphiuma	$\frac{1}{363}$
Proteus	$\frac{1}{400}$
Siren	$\frac{1}{420}$
Menopoma	$\frac{1}{563}$

FISHES.

Pike	$\frac{1}{2000}$
Perch	$\frac{1}{2460}$
Lamprey	$\frac{1}{2134}$

It must be admitted, therefore, that while the red blood-corpuscles of the mammalia can be shown by measurement to differ in size (see table), the blood examined being freshly drawn in each instance, red blood-corpuscles as obtained from blood-stains cannot be positively identified by such a method as human red blood-corpuscles. Any evidence offered as positive proof based upon micrometric methods that blood is human, as distinguished from other mammalian blood, must be regarded as only circumstantial at best, for the following three reasons mentioned above: (1) The micrometric method is approximative. (2) The size of the corpuscle restored is variable, depending upon the amount of fluid absorbed. (3) The size of the corpuscles varies, even in the blood of the same mammal.

Recently an attempt has been made to distinguish human blood from that of other mammals by dissolving dried coagula in a suitable medium and staining the granules of the white corpuscles or leucocytes. It is claimed that the leucocytes are more resistant to the disintegrating influence of drying and redissolving than the red corpuscles; that the granules of the leucocytes of the blood differ in man and animals not only as regards their size, but in the manner in which they are affected by staining materials, some of the granules—about 3 per cent.—in human blood staining only with acid—"acidophiles"; others—97 per cent.— with neither acid nor basic material, but only with particular combination "triacid" stains—"neutrophiles"; that neutrophiles are found in the blood of "apes" and acidophiles and non-granuliferous leucocytes in the blood of the remaining mammals.* While this method may prove of service in the future as a means of distinguishing human blood from that of other mammals, as no cases have occurred as yet *in foro*, at least so far as is known to the author, by which the value of the method could be practically tested, it would be premature upon his part to express any opinion as to its merits.

The red blood-corpuscles of man and the mammalia generally can be readily distinguished, however, from those of birds, reptiles, and fishes, the latter being not only relatively of large size, but oval in form and nucleated (Fig.

---

* Walker, Ernest L.: "A New Method of Distinguishing Human from Other Mammalian Blood in Medico-legal Cases," Harvard Medical School, Boston, 1900. The author does not say whether by "apes" he refers to the anthropoids or to ordinary monkeys.

18). It should be mentioned, in this connection, that the red corpuscles of the camel and llama are oval, and that those of the lamprey are somewhat circular. No difficulty

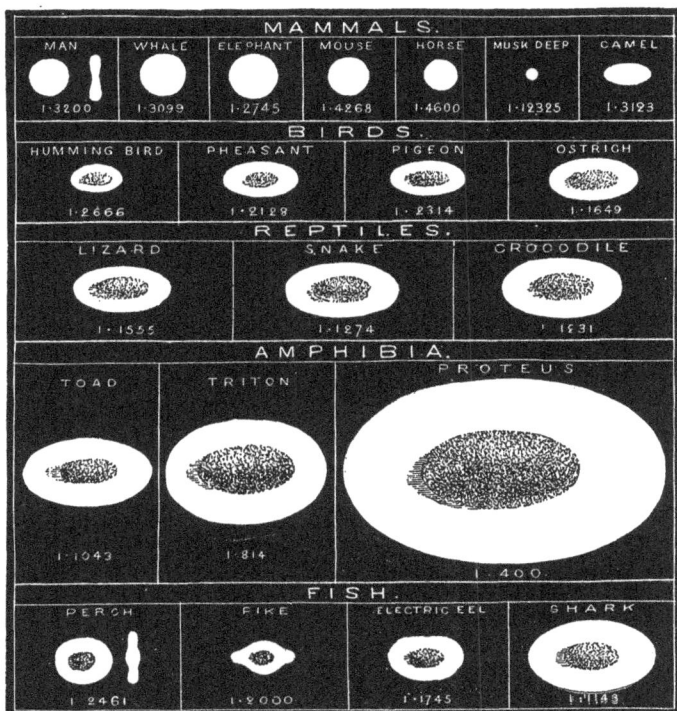

Fig. 18.—Blood-corpuscles of vertebrates.

should arise on account of this circumstance, for, as in the case of the camelidæ, the corpuscles are without a nucleus, though ovoid in form; while in the lamprey the corpuscles are nucleated, even if circular. The fact that the red corpuscle of a bird differs in form and in size from that of a mammal is very important from a medico-legal point of view.

Thus, for example, a woman accused of murdering her child accounted for the blood found on some clothing by stating that it was fowl's blood. The blood, on examination, was shown not to be fowl's blood, the corpuscles being neither oval nor nucleated, but round and unnucleated. While the medical examiner was unable to state positively that the blood was human blood, he at least convicted the woman of having lied, and thereby materially weakened the defense. In a similar instance, in which a woman was found murdered, the explanation offered by the man accused of the crime was that the blood spilled in the wagon was that of a chicken which had been killed by him for market. It was shown, however, by the medical expert, that the red blood-corpuscles obtained from the blood were round and without nucleus. That testimony alone proved that the statement of the defendant was false, and was in itself presumptive evidence of guilt and ultimately led to the confession of the crime, and to conviction and execution. In another case, among the circumstances that led to the suspicion that a man found dead with severe bruises on the head had been murdered, was the finding, on the trousers of the suspected murderer, of a large spot of blood, the presence of which the defendant tried to explain away by saying that it was the blood of a fowl. The blood was shown, however, to be that of a mammal—probably of man, but positively not that of a bird.*

Poachers, in getting their clothing stained with blood in fights with gamekeepers, often resulting in murder, have

* Taylor: *op. cit.*, p. 289.

tried to account for the blood in a similar way by saying that it was that of partridges or pheasants.

Blood-crystals, due to the crystallization of hæmoglobin or its modifications, constitute an important proof of the existence of blood.* The hæmoglobin-crystals can be readily obtained from freshly drawn human blood by evaporating a drop of the blood to dryness on a glass slide,

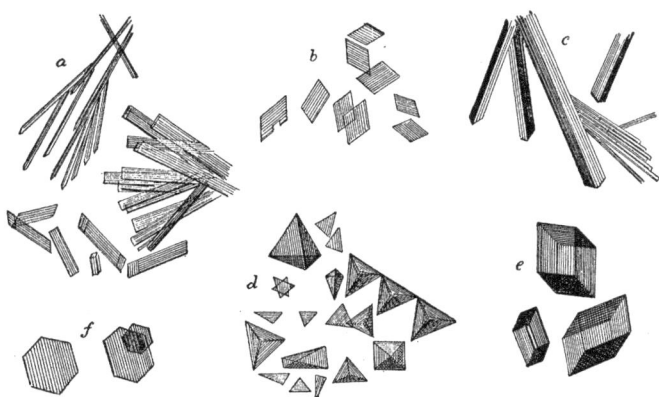

Fig. 19.—Blood-crystals: *a,* Human blood-crystals (hæmoglobin); *b,* human blood-crystals (hæmatin hydrochlorate); *c,* human blood-crystals (hæmatin); *d,* crystals from guinea-pig's blood; *e,* from horse's blood; *f,* from squirrel's blood.

adding a drop of distilled water, and allowing the water to evaporate under a thin glass cover. The glass slide having been transferred to the stage of the microscope, the crystals will soon appear in various forms and sizes, but usually as small prisms (Fig. 19, *a*). If the blood submitted for examination has, however, undergone changes, the hæmoglobin ($C_{636}H_{1025}N_{164}FeS_3O_{181}$) having been converted into hæmatin

* Preyer: "Die Blut-Crystalle," Jena, 1871; Dragendorf in Maschka, vol. I, S. 483.

($C_{32}H_{32}N_4O_4Fe$), as would have occurred in the formation of an old blood-clot, a very convenient method of obtaining that substance in the form of crystals is to mix together on a watch-glass a drop of blood, or of the solution of the suspected substance, with glacial acetic acid in excess, and slowly evaporate to dryness over a spirit-lamp. The mass so obtained, when viewed under the microscope, will usually exhibit the crystals in great numbers (Fig. 19, c).

In order, however, to obtain from dried blood, crystals of hæmatin hydrochlorate, formerly known as hæmin ($C_{32}H_{30}N_4FeO_3HCl$), the suspected material should be placed

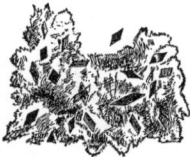

Fig. 20. — Blood - crystals (hæmatin hydrochlorate).

upon a glass slide and moistened with a solution of sodium chloride (1 grain of salt to 4 ounces of distilled water) and covered with a large thin cover-glass, under the edge of which glacial acetic acid is allowed to run. The liquid should then be heated to dryness at a boiling temperature, the slide allowed to cool, and the material placed under the microscope, the crystals soon appearing. Another method of obtaining crystals of hæmatin hydrochlorate is to triturate the substance suspected to be blood in a mortar with a little common salt, add glacial acetic acid, and warm the mixture till bubbles appear, and then set aside to cool. On transforming the material so treated to the field of the microscope, crystals will be usually found in great number. Crystals of hæmatin hydrochlorate, or Teichmann's crystals, as obtained by either of the two methods just described, when viewed under the microscope appear as minute flat rhomboids (Fig. 19, b, Fig. 20), lying in many cases superimposed in the form of crosses or in the form of stars. They vary in size from the $\frac{1}{6000}$ to the $\frac{1}{1200}$ of an inch in length, and in color from a clear yellow to a reddish-brown. The determination of a substance to be blood, by the developing from it of Teichmann's crystals by the methods just described, is a most delicate one. Indeed, from as small a quantity as the $\frac{1}{500}$ to the $\frac{1}{1000}$ of a grain of dried blood crystals of hæmatin hydrochlorate can be obtained and the presence of blood thereby satisfactorily demonstrated. This test for proving the presence of blood is not only of the greatest practical value to the medical jurist on account of its delicacy, but from the fact that, notwithstanding that the blood may have been spilled many years before examination, or washed, rubbed, fouled, discolored, or decomposed, nevertheless, as some of its coloring-matter usually remains, the obtaining of the crystals in most cases is made possible. For example, Büchner and Simon proved the existence of blood in a small rag cut from a butcher's slaughtering trousers, which had been in use for eight years, though not worn for a year and a half previously.* In the year 1819 Kotzebue was assassinated by Sand in his own house, the papers upon his desk being stained with his blood. In 1879, sixty years afterward, crystals of hæmatin hydrochlorate were readily obtained from these stains, thereby proving that they had been made by blood.† While the presence of such crystals undoubtedly proves that the material from which they were obtained was blood, unfortunately their presence does not necessarily prove that

* "Archiv f. patholog. Anat. u. Physiologie," neue Folge, Bd. vi, 2. Heft, 1858, S. 50.

† "A System of Legal Medicine," by A. McLane Hamilton, M.D., and Lawrence Godkin, Esq., vol. i, New York, 1894, p. 163.

it was human blood, for while the crystals of the blood of the guinea-pig (Fig. 19, d), squirrel, etc. (Fig. 19, f), differ in form from those of man, the crystals of the blood of some mammals (Fig. 19, e) are indistinguishable from those of the former. Therefore, the presence of blood-crystals as evidence that a suspected material from which they have been obtained is positively human blood is of but little more value from a medico-legal point of view than the presence of blood-corpuscles.

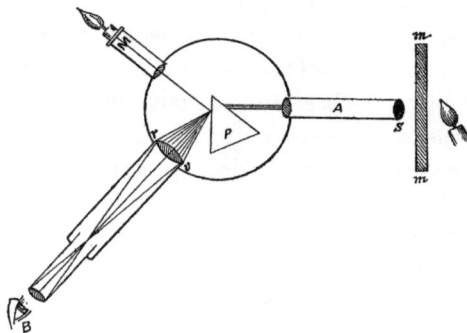

Fig. 21.—Layer of blood in a glass vessel through which the light is transmitted; scheme of a spectroscope for observing the spectrum of blood: A, Tube; S, slit; m m, layer of blood with flame in front of it; P, prism; M, scale; B, eye of observer looking through a telescope; r v, spectrum.

The **spectroscopic method** of investigating blood-stains is based upon the fact that blood interferes with the transmission of certain rays of light, and that it gives rise to what are known as the dark absorption bands of the blood spectrum. It is well known that when sunlight is transmitted through a prism it is decomposed into the seven colors: violet, indigo, blue, green, yellow, orange, red (Plate 1, Fig. 1). If, however, a weak solution of arterial blood—that is, of blood containing a small amount of oxyhæmoglobin—be placed in a suitable glass vessel (Fig.

21, M), between the source of light and the prism, two
dark bands will appear in that part of the solar spectrum
(Plate 1, Fig. 4) previously occupied by the yellow-green,
and more particularly in that portion of the yellow adjoin-
ing the orange and yellow-green, the two dark bands being
separated by that part of the yellow light still transmitted
through the blood. If the solution of hæmoglobin be,
however, concentrated, the two bands are replaced by
one broad band (Plate 1, Fig. 3); and if still more concentrated, all the light is absorbed except that of the
red and orange (Plate 1, Fig. 2). If, on the contrary,
the solution be very weak, but one narrow band will
appear. If the arterial blood be now replaced by venous
blood, or simply deoxidized,—that is, the oxyhæmoglobin
converted into hæmoglobin, as can be done by adding
a reducing agent having an avidity for oxygen such as
ammonium sulphid,—the two dark bands will disappear,
and in that part of the spectrum where the yellow light
was transmitted there will appear one dark band, while
that part of the spectrum lying on either side of the dark
band will be occupied by the yellow and green (Plate 1,
Fig. 6). By simply shaking the solution with air the
hæmoglobin is re-oxidized, becomes again oxyhæmoglobin,
and gives, as before, the spectrum of arterial blood with
two bands (Plate 1, Fig. 6).

It is true that solutions of the coloring-matter of
the petals of cineraria,* of cochineal, madder, and other
red dyes present dark bands in their spectrum, but their
situation is either not exactly the same as those of the

* Of the different menstrua used by the writer to obtain the coloring-matter from the petals of cineraria, glacial acetic acid was found
to be the best.

7

blood spectrum, or they can be distinguished from those
of the latter by the action of ammonia and potassium sulphate.

The spectroscope employed in medico-legal examinations
is the same as that used in chemical and physical researches,
the essential parts being shown in figure 21, or it may consist simply of a spectroscopic attachment to a microscope.
By means of the spectroscope, not only can blood be shown
to be present, but arterial or venous blood can be distinguished from blood that has absorbed carbon monoxid gas
(Plate 1, Fig. 7), and from solutions of acid and alkali
hæmatin (Plate 1, Figs. 9, 10), the dark bands presented
by their spectra being respectively different in each instance.

The delicacy of the spectroscopic method of investigating
fresh blood is such that a solution containing one grain of
oxyhæmoglobin, upon which the absorption of the light
depends, to a pint of water will interfere with the transmission of strong sunlight sufficiently to render the two dark
bands visible.

In cases of carbon monoxid poisoning, where the corpuscles absorb the gas with even greater avidity than oxygen,
and hold it with greater tenacity, the spectrum gives two
bands (Plate 1, Fig. 7) which differ, however, sufficiently
in position from those due to oxyhæmoglobin as to be distinguishable from the latter. When blood has only been
exposed a sufficiently long time for the hæmoglobin to have
been converted into methæmoglobin, which appears to
differ from oxyhæmoglobin only in its oxygen being held
in more stable combination, the spectrum gives three
bands, two like those of carbon monoxid and one situated
in the orange part of the spectrum (Plate 1, Fig. 8).   The

spectrum of acid hæmatin produced through the decomposition of oxyhæmoglobin by acids gives one narrow band situated in the orange-red end of the spectrum (Plate 1, Fig. 9). In cases where the oxyhæmoglobin has been converted by long exposure or by washing with soap and water, etc., into hæmatin, which is insoluble in pure water, it will be necessary to treat the suspected material with citric acid or ammonia in order to dissolve the coloring-matter, and in some cases even a moderate heat must be applied as well. The solution so obtained, as from a linen rag, pieces of leather, wood, iron, etc., on being transferred, after dilution, if necessary, to the glass vessel attached to the spectroscope (Plate 1, Fig. 10), will give one broad band situated in the orange of the spectrum. Alkali hæmatin, like oxyhæmoglobin, is susceptible of being reduced, or deoxidized, and reoxidized again. The spectrum of reduced hæmatin, or hæmochromogen, as it is also called, gives two absorption bands—a broad one situated in the yellow, and a narrow one in the green part of the spectrum.*

The spectroscopic method is the most convenient, reliable, and delicate of the different methods which have been described for investigating blood-stains, it enabling the medical examiner to state positively that stains years old on wood, linen, or iron, even when found in a putrid condition, were made by blood. Thus, according to Sorby, a spot of blood the $\frac{1}{10}$ of an inch in diameter, the coloring-matter of which amounted to only the $\frac{1}{1000}$

---

* A convenient method of showing the absorption bands to a large audience is to project the solar spectrum upon a white surface and then interpose between the beam of light and the prism the solution of blood.

of a grain sufficed to prove conclusively the presence of blood when examined spectroscopically. Blood was detected by the same high authority, in the form of deoxidized hæmatin on the rusty blade of a knife with which a murder had been committed, after a lapse of ten years.* The spectrum of hæmatin was obtained by Tidy from stains on the clothing preserved by the relatives of an officer said to have been killed in battle in 1771, and therefore after a lapse of more than one hundred years.† The spectroscopic method of investigating blood-stains,

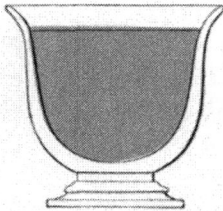

Fig. 22.—Blood before coagulation.   Fig. 23.—Blood-clot floating in the fluid serum after coagulation.

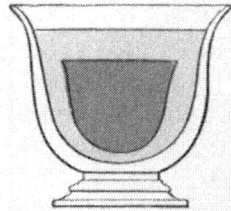

reliable and delicate though it may be, unfortunately does not enable the examiner to state that a suspected material is human blood, but only that it is blood. By none of the methods, therefore, of examining blood-stains, whether chemical, microscopic, or spectroscopic, can human blood be distinguished positively from that of other animals.

Coagulation of Blood.—One of the most remarkable properties of the blood is its power of separating into clot and serum, due to the coagulation and subsequent shrinkage of its fibrin (Figs. 22, 23), the process being com-

* Taylor: *op. cit.*, p. 283.   † Tidy: *op. cit.*, part i, p. 217.

pleted outside the body within a period of from ten to twelve hours.

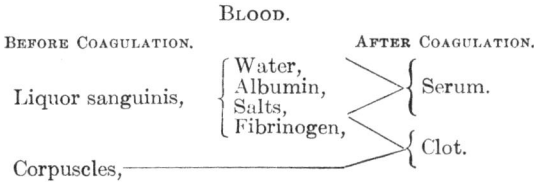

BLOOD.

BEFORE COAGULATION.		AFTER COAGULATION.
Liquor sanguinis,	{ Water, Albumin, Salts, Fibrinogen,	} Serum.
Corpuscles,		{ Clot.

Conditions Influencing Coagulation of Blood.—
While the blood does not usually coagulate in the living body, it almost invariably does so in the dead body, and within a period varying between twelve and twenty-four hours. There are various conditions which influence the coagulation of the blood within and without the body, some of which are better understood than others. Only those conditions influencing coagulation which may have an importance from a medico-legal point of view need be here considered. Blood flowing from a small orifice coagulates more quickly than when flowing from a large one; more quickly when it is received into a shallow, rough vessel than when in a deep, smooth one. The coagulation of the blood is retarded when mixed with solutions of sodium sulphate and carbonate, and prevented by the addition of potassium oxalate. Rapid freezing will prevent the coagulation of the blood; blood so frozen will, however, coagulate if carefully thawed. This is of importance practically, since in a case that came under the observation of the author the fact of some frozen material coagulating after it was thawed led to its further examination and to ultimately proving that the frozen material was blood. A temperature of from 32° to 140° F. favors coagulation.

The menstrual blood is kept in a more or less fluid condition by the vaginal secretions.

Amount of Blood in the Body.—The medical expert is often asked to express an opinion as to how much blood the body of the deceased contained. While it is impossible to state exactly how much blood there is in any human body, it may be said that on an average there is one pound of blood for every eight pounds of body-weight; that is, there would be about sixteen pounds of blood in the body of a man weighing one hundred and twenty-eight pounds. This estimate is based upon the fact that twelve pounds of blood were collected during an execution by beheading of a criminal weighing one hundred and twenty-eight pounds, and that four pounds of blood were obtained after the execution by washing out the blood-vessels.*

* Lehmann: "Lehrbuch der phys. Chemie," 1852, Bd. ii, S. 234.

CHAPTER VI.

Death from Burns and Scalds—Spontaneous Combustion—Heat and Cold—Lightning—Starvation.

Burns and Scalds.—A burn may be defined, medico-legally, as an injury produced by the application of a heated substance to the surface of the body, while a scald results from the application of a liquid at about its boiling-point.

While neither burns nor scalds are regarded in law as wounds, they are included, in the statute of wounding, among the bodily injuries dangerous to life.* The effects of burns and scalds upon the body are essentially the same. Burns vary in their intensity from a mere redness of the skin to a complete carbonization of the body.

The danger from burns depends more on their extent than upon their depth. This is due to the fact that the excretory and heat-regulating functions of the skin are interfered with in proportion to the extent of the skin involved.

It may be stated, as a general rule, that if one-third of the body, or even one-third of the skin, be severely burned, the burn will *probably* prove fatal. Death in the case of burns is usually due to shock, though often caused by suffocation, exhaustion, or gangrene. It must be remembered, however, that the result of burns will

* Taylor: *op. cit.*, p. 390; Tidy: *op. cit.*, p. 453.

be very much influenced by the age and constitution of the individual and the part of the body affected. Thus, for example, burns are more dangerous in the young than in the old; more so on the trunk of the body than on the limbs; more so if in separate patches than when continuous, supposing the parts burned are of equal extent.

The post-mortem appearances observed in cases of death from burns are not very constant. Among those frequently noticed, however, are capillary injection of the mucous membrane of the alimentary canal and bronchi, perforating ulcers of stomach and duodenum, and serious effusion of the ventricles of the brain.

As cases have occurred in which the body of a person murdered has been burned after death, in the hope that the death might be attributed to accident, and so enable the murderer to escape the consequences of his crime, it is most important that the medical examiner should be able to state whether a body was burned during life or after death. Thus, in the case of the Countess of Goerlitz, who was found dead and burned in her room at Darmstadt, it was held by some of the physicians that the deceased had not been murdered by one Stauff, as many suspected, but had died of spontaneous combustion. The facts of the case having been referred to Liebig and Bischoff, those distinguished authorities reported that in their opinion the woman had been murdered and the body burnt after death for the purpose of concealing the crime. After conviction Stauff confessed that the Countess had entered the room as he was committing a robbery; that he strangled her, placed her dead body in a chair, around which he placed the combustible articles of the furniture, and then set fire to them, hoping in this way to destroy the proofs of his crime.*

As an illustration of the importance of a careful examination being made of the bodies of persons found dead and burnt, it may be mentioned that in one instance where the bodies of six persons were found dead in a house that had been burnt, death, in the opinion of the medical examiner, was attributed to the fire and the bodies were buried. Some time after, suspicion being excited on account of a murder being committed near the house, the bodies were disinterred and, after a careful examination, death was shown to have been caused by blows inflicted probably with a hatchet, which was subsequently shown to be the case, one man having murdered all six persons in this way.

Vesication.—Among the facts that may be mentioned as proving that burns had been inflicted during life, a most important one is the presence of blisters, and particularly of blisters containing serum, a blister being due to the exudation of the serum of the blood from the surface of the true skin and its collection between the latter and the cuticle. It is true that blisters may be produced a few minutes after death by heat, but when so produced they contain air, not serum.†

In dropsical persons blisters can also be produced after death by the application of heat, but the serum found in them is invariably thin and watery, rarely tinged with blood, and giving only a trace of albumin.‡

On the other hand, the absence of blisters does not

* Taylor: *op. cit.*, p. 394.
† Christison: " Edinburgh Medical Journal," 1831, p. 320.
‡ Tidy: *op. cit.*, part I, p. 482.

prove that a body was not burned during life, since blisters do not necessarily result from burns. Further, blisters, even when present, are sometimes so modified by the effects of the heat when intense as to be unrecognizable.

The bullæ produced by putrefaction are occasionally mistaken by the superficial observer for blisters caused by burns. The green discoloration of the skin present in putrefaction, together with the absence of both a reddish state of the skin and the line of redness separating the dead white skin surrounding the blister from the part of the skin unaffected by the heat, will usually enable the observer to distinguish the one from the other.

The Line of Redness.—The red line just referred to is not only found surrounding the blisters that are caused by burns, but in their absence as well, between the dry, coppery red, parchment-like skin, that has been burnt, and the healthy part; the red color of the line fading away into that of the surrounding skin. The red line persists after death; it does not disappear under pressure, and it cannot be produced by the application of heat to the living body. The red line, being due to vital action, its presence indicating, as it does, the demarcation between the living tissue that was destroyed by the burn and the part that escaped, is a most positive proof that the burn was inflicted during life or at least within a few minutes after somatic death—*i. e.*, during the period when molecular life persists.* Indeed, in the case of burns the presence of blisters and the red line is so

* That molecular life persists at least for some time after the somatic death appears to be shown from the fact of hairs and nails growing, and glands secreting, after the general death of the body.

important that in the opinion of the highest authorities *
it is impossible to mistake a burn inflicted during life
for one inflicted after death. On the other hand, the
absence of blisters and of the red line would not necessarily
prove that the burn had been inflicted after death, since,
as already mentioned, blisters are not invariably formed
by burns; and the red line being due to vital action and
requiring time for its formation, the death might be so
sudden as not to permit of this.

It must be admitted, however, that in those cases
where the body has been roasted or charred, it would
be impossible to say whether the body had been burnt
before or after death, since a living body can neither be
roasted nor charred; that is to say, that the roasting or
charring would not commence until after the death of
the individual, even supposing that the fire had been
applied to the body primarily before death. On the
other hand, the presence of granulations ("proud flesh"),
pus, or gangrene, in the burnt parts—essentially vital
products—may be regarded as positive proof that the
person had lived for some time after the infliction of the
burn.

Difference of opinion still prevails among medical
jurists as to the propriety of administering opium in
cases of persons suffering from burns, it being alleged
that the coma produced by the drug might be attributed to the burn.† Indeed, in a well-known case where
a surgeon was charged with the manslaughter of a child
by giving opium, his acquittal was largely due to the

---

* Orfila: "Méd. Légale," 1821, t. I, p. 457; Devergie: "Méd.
Légale," 1836, p. 273; Casper: op. cit., vol. I, p. 302.

† Taylor: op. cit., p. 390; Tidy: op. cit., part I, p. 464.

testimony of the celebrated Abernethy, which was to the effect that the practice of giving opium in such cases was proper, and that the coma resulted from the burn and not from the opium. In the judgment of the author at least, the first duty of the physician is to his patient— to relieve pain, to save life, to administer any drug by which these objects will be best attained, utterly irrespective of any consideration as to the question of the future determination of the innocence or guilt of the person accused of having inflicted the injuries from which the patient suffers.

Spontaneous Combustion.—As this subject has just been referred to in connection with the case of the Countess of Goerlitz, and as death is still attributed in some cases to such a cause by ignorant, credulous people, and even by some otherwise scientific writers, it may as well be mentioned that, so far as the author has been able to learn, there is no authentic case of true spontaneous combustion of the human body on record. In the case, however, of habitual drunkards, especially if corpulent, the body appears to be highly inflammable and readily set on fire, as by the upsetting of a candle, a spark from the fire, which under the circumstances might readily lead to its ignition and ultimate destruction by combustion.

The cases of so-called spontaneous combustion that have been reported from time to time as occurring in man, when thoroughly sifted and freed from miraculous details, can be very well accounted for in this way.

Death from Heat and Cold.—Death from heat does not, as a general rule, become a subject of medico-legal investigation. As, however, in cases of death from sunstroke, from exposure to the heat of engine-rooms, etc., doubts may be raised at the coroner's inquest, especially in the absence of witnesses, as to whether death was really due to such causes, and was not suicidal or homicidal, it is important that the medical examiner should be familiar with the symptoms and post-mortem changes presented in such cases. The symptoms of exposure to excessive heat, whether to that of the direct rays of the sun, or to that of the peculiar atmosphere of the engine-rooms and factories, saturated with moisture, and therefore interfering with the heat-regulating functions of the skin, vary from headache with drowsiness to complete insensibility, coma, and paralysis. In most such cases death appears to be due to paralysis of the heart. Among the post-mortem appearances which are not constant may be mentioned congestion of the brain and its membranes, serum in the ventricles, congestion of the heart, lungs, and viscera. In some cases, however, there is anæmia of the brain.

Death from cold is usually accidental, occurring, for example, in drunkards who have fallen asleep in the snow, or in persons who have lost their way in woods or in snow-drifts. Death from cold is, however, not infrequently homicidal. Thus, newly born infants are often intentionally frozen to death by exposure to the air of a very cold winter night. Death takes place very quickly under such circumstances, infants having but little power to resist cold. Young children have been frozen by being immersed in vessels of ice-water. Lunatics have died of exhaustion after too long exposure to the cold shower-bath administered as a punishment for misbehavior. In all such cases the temperature of the air, the season of the year, the time of day, the place of exposure, must be all taken into consideration by the examiner.

The post-mortem changes in death from cold are not characteristic. Among the most noticeable are the general pallor and stiffness of the body, the irregular and diffused red patches on different parts of the body, even in such as are not dependent, the unusual accumulation of blood on both sides of the heart, and the congestion of the viscera. In all cases of death supposed to be due to cold, it is important to determine whether the body, when found, was putrefying, since, as putrefaction is prevented by freezing, it would be a strong proof, if a body were found putrefied in ice or snow, that death was not due to freezing, but that the freezing had occurred after death.

Death by Lightning.—Death by lightning is of medico-legal interest from the fact that in the case of bodies found dead in remote places and bearing marks of violence death has been attributed to murder rather than to lightning. The effects of death from lightning vary considerably in their intensity. Frequently the hair is singed, the skin deeply burned or punctured, the clothes burned, the boots torn open. If such articles as watch-chains, or coins, or knives happen to constitute part of the circuit, they will be usually found melted or half melted. In some cases the body may be uninjured, and yet the clothes burned or entirely torn off. In other cases the clothes may entirely escape, and yet the body may be much burned. In death from lightning the brain and its membranes are usually found congested, the brain being frequently disorganized. The stomach, intestines, and liver are usually congested. The heart does not present any marked alteration. The lungs are, however, usually congested and full of mucus.

Rigor mortis frequently sets in immediately after death. In such cases the body is found in exactly the same attitudê as when it was struck. The coagulation of the blood is retarded. On the other hand, putrefaction is accelerated.

Death by lightning is usually instantaneous, being due to shock. But in some cases death is delayed, being then due to some affection of the brain or spinal cord, such as epilepsy, paralysis, effusion of blood, tetanus, etc. The effect of a stroke of lightning, as is well known, is very capricious. Of three or four persons sitting under a tree, one or two only may be killed, the others escaping. Persons are reported as having been killed while sitting under a low tree, notwithstanding the presence of tall trees, a lightning rod, and an iron bridge near by. Should the question ever arise as to whether death was due to a stroke of lightning, such facts as there having been a thunderstorm at about the supposed period of death, the peculiar appearance of the deceased, the co-existence of burns and wounds, the finding of half-melted buttons and coins, would strongly point to that conclusion.*

Death from Starvation.—The symptoms of and postmortem appearances in death from starvation, whether the system be deprived suddenly or gradually of food, are essentially the same. Advantage is often taken of

* For post-mortem appearances presented in cases of death by electrocution or from the accidental application of electricity, see Taylor, *op. cit.*, p. 470; Richardson: "Medical Times and Gazette," May 15, 1869, p. 511; Allan McLane Hamilton: "System of Legal Medicine," New York, 1894, vol. I, p. 134; vol. II, p. 367. Bullard: "The Medico-Legal Relations of Electricity," "Medical Jurisprudence, Forensic Medicine, and Toxicology," by R. A. Witthaus and Tracy C. Becker, vol. II, New York, 1894.

this fact by those in charge of so-called "baby-farms," where, to save expense, infants are slowly starved by food insufficient in quantity and quality, and where their death is attributed to the diseases common to infancy. Usually, in such cases, the true cause of death is overlooked, suspicion even being averted, as the length of time is so great that months often elapse before death is accomplished by the starving process. For this reason death from chronic starvation is so much more common than from acute starvation. Indeed, death from acute starvation occurs almost always accidentally, as in the case of those who are buried in a mine, or of those who are shipwrecked or lost on desert wastes. Starvation is very rarely suicidal. Lunatics and prisoners sometimes attempt to take their own lives by abstaining wholly from food, but, as a general rule, such attempts are unsuccessful.

Among the symptoms of starvation may be mentioned severe pain in the epigastrium, which usually passes away in a day or so, being replaced by an indescribable feeling of weakness, a sort of sinking. The face becomes pale and cadaverous, and there is a wild look in the eye. General emaciation follows, and an offensive odor is noticed about the body, which is covered with a brownish secretion. The voice becomes weak, and muscular effort impossible. The intelligence can, with difficulty, be aroused. Immediately before death there is a decided fall in the temperature. Death takes place usually in from ten to twelve days, often accompanied with mania and convulsions. In death from starvation the most important changes noticed on post-mortem examination are the loss in body-weight, the almost entire absence of fat and blood, and the loss in bulk of the most important viscera. The coats of the intestines are so thinned as to be almost transparent, the gall-bladder is distended with bile, and decomposition sets in very readily. As already mentioned, death from inanition or chronic starvation is characterized by the symptoms and post-mortem changes just described as resulting in death from acute starvation.

It is often stated that the quantity of food required by a healthy man doing work during twenty-four hours is as follows:

Meat,	16 oz.
Bread,	19 "
Butter or fat,	3½ "
Water,	52 fl. oz.

If health, however, is to be maintained, fresh vegetables, fruits, tea, coffee, and sugar should be added from time to time to the above diet.

8

CHAPTER VII.

Death from Suffocation—By Strangulation—By Hanging—Drowning.

Death from Suffocation.—Death from suffocation, whether by strangulation, hanging, or drowning, or however produced, is due in each instance to the same cause—the deprivation of the system of air, or asphyxia.

The post-mortem appearances observed in such cases are usually lividity of the face and lips, congestion of the eyes, bloody mucous froth about the mouth and nose, congestion of the lungs and of the right side of the heart and kidneys. Apart from the three principal modes of death from suffocation, just referred to, and which will be considered separately, there are other modes of death from suffocation, in which air is excluded, not by extensive pressure on the trachea, as in strangulation or hanging, but as in drowning, and in other cases in which the nostrils and mouth only are closed, and which, occurring so frequently, demand some attention. Thus, for example, infants are frequently suffocated accidentally from being too closely wrapped up, or from being rolled upon by their mothers, often so intoxicated as to be unaware of what they are doing, and who in extenuation say that the child slept in the same bed and on waking it was found dead.

Children, feeble persons, and drunkards have been suffocated by falling into ash-heaps, dirt-piles, etc. The

passage into the larynx of marbles and whistles accidentally swallowed by children, of half-chewed meat
bolted through over-haste in eating,—a habit unfortunately
too common even in adults,—is a not uncommon cause
of suffocation.* The fact that food may be accidentally
impacted in the larynx illustrates the importance of a
careful examination always being made of the air-passages
in cases of suspected murder. Thus, in a case that occurred
at Hillingdon, England, a man was accused of the murder of
another, it being in evidence that the two had been fighting, that both had fallen to the ground, and that they were
finally separated. Two hours after the struggle the
deceased was stated to have left the dinner table and
was found outside of the cottage, leaning against the
latter, as if in a falling position, where he expired in two
or three minutes. Death being attributed by the medical
examiner to apoplexy induced by the violence, the person
with whom the deceased had been fighting was arrested
on the charge of manslaughter. The coroner insisting,
however, upon the mouth and throat being examined,
which the medical examiner had neglected to do, death
was shown to have been really caused by suffocation
due to the food just eaten having been drawn into the
larynx, completely plugging the latter, and the defendant
was discharged.†

Occasionally, suffocation is intentionally produced, as
in cases where individuals, having determined to commit
suicide, force foreign bodies, like balls of hay or cotton,
for example, down their own throats. Thus, in the case

---

* Tidy: *op. cit.*, part ii, pp. 448, 449; Taylor: *op. cit.*, p. 426;
Wharton and Stillé: vol. iii, p. 348.

† "Lancet," 1850, i, p. 313.

of a woman whose death was at first attributed to apoplexy, it was shown subsequently in the dissecting-room that death was really due to suffocation caused by spindle cotton, which the deceased, when confined in prison, had with suicidal intent forced down her throat, completely plugging the latter.*

Death from suffocation may be, however, homicidal as well as accidental or suicidal. Indeed, one of the commonest ways of killing new-born children is by suffocation, the crime being easily committed and leaving but few traces to tell the tale. Frequently, persons have been suffocated by having foreign bodies like corks and pieces of meat forced down their throats, the murderers hoping that death would be attributed to accidental suffocation, and thus have suspicion diverted from themselves.

In the case of a woman found dead with a cork in the larynx, for example, it was suggested that the deceased had drawn the cork with her teeth and that it had been accidentally sucked into the larynx. This view was, however, inconsistent with the fact that the sealed end of the cork was found uppermost, and which proved, according to the medical examiner, that the cork had been forced down the woman's throat when in a helpless state of intoxication. Five persons were known to have been present with the deceased at the time of her death, but as it was impossible to fix with any certainty upon the person who had committed the crime, the man on whom the strongest suspicion fell was acquitted, the verdict being "not proven."† On the other hand, a Russian sentry being found dead in his watch-box with

---

* " Edinburgh Med. and Surg. Journal," 1842, p. 391.
† Taylor: *op. cit.*, p. 451.

a large piece of meat in his pharynx, pressing upon and closing the larynx, death was supposed to have been accidental. As a matter of fact, however, his superior officer confessed to having suffocated the man and then placed the meat in his throat to divert suspicion.* The medical examiner, in cases of death from suffocation, even after most careful examination, should be extremely cautious, therefore, in expressing an opinion as to whether death was accidental, suicidal, or homicidal.

Death from Suffocation by Strangulation.—Strangulation may be produced either by simple pressure of the hand on the windpipe, as in throttling, or by means of a rope, strap, handkerchief, piece of a sheet, bowstring, etc. Among the signs of death from strangulation may be mentioned the staring eyes with dilated pupils, the livid and swollen face, the protruding and often-bitten tongue, blood about the nose, mouth, and ears, turgidity of the genitalia, with escape of urine and feces. The larynx is flattened, congested internally, and coated over with a bloody frothy mucus. The right side of the heart and the venous system are gorged with blood. The marks made by the fingers and thumb upon the front of the neck, as in throttling, or the horizontal mark or marks made by the cord according to the number of times it was wound around the neck, with the infiltrated blood beneath, are striking evidences of death from strangulation, and which in some cases persist weeks and even years after burial.

It must be admitted, nevertheless, that, according to Tidy,† an ecchymosed mark can be produced experimentally within three hours, a non-ecchymosed one within six

* Tidy: *op. cit.*, part ii, p. 462. † Tidy: *op. cit.*, part ii, p. 431.

hours, after death, while Casper * states, as the result
of his experiments, "that any ligature with which any
body may be suspended or strangled, not only within
a few hours, but even days after death, especially if the
body be forcibly pulled downward, may produce a mark
precisely similar to that which is observed in most of
those hanged while alive." Indeed, as death caused by
either strangling or hanging is so sudden that the mark
of the cord can only be produced after death, the latter
must be regarded as a "purely cadaveric phenomenon."

While no doubt it is true that such marks can be made
by winding a cord around the neck of a dead body, and
that therefore too much importance must not be attached
to their presence, it must be borne in mind that as the
livid, swollen countenance, the protruded tongue, the
staring eyeballs, always present in death from strangulation, cannot be produced after death, the former must
be always taken into consideration, as well as the marks
observed on the front of the neck.

> " But see his face is black and full of blood,
>   His eyeballs further out than when he lived,
>   Staring full ghastly like a strangled man,
>   His hair up-reared, his nostrils stretched with struggling;
>   His hands abroad displayed as one that grasped
>   And tugged for life and was by strength subdued."

Strangulation differs from hanging principally in the
position of the cord, which is horizontal in the former
case and oblique in the latter. From a medico-legal point
of view this is an important distinction, since death from
strangulation would be usually regarded as homicidal,
that from hanging as suicidal, though not necessarily,

* Casper: *op. cit.*, vol. II, p. 173.

since there are a sufficient number of well-attested cases
on record * to prove that persons can voluntarily destroy themselves by strangulation even though it seems
apparently impossible. As an illustration of such cases
may be mentioned that of the Italian Pozzala, a por-
ter found dead in the attic of the house of his em-
ployer with a piece of ordinary sash line coiled four times
around his neck, two of the coils being so tight as to
make it difficult to undo them, one end of the line being
held by the right hand, the other by the left, with a turn
of the line around each hand, evidently to hold it more
securely. The general appearance of the deceased and
the results of the post-mortem examination were such as
are usually found in deaths from strangulation, and
the evidence was such that in the opinion of the coroner
there was no doubt but that death was suicidal.†

Suicidal strangulation is rare. Among the insane it
sometimes occurs, being so easily accomplished. Indeed,
in certain cases it requires the greatest vigilance on the
part of the attendants to prevent it. In one instance, for
example, where a gentleman had been placed in a private insane asylum, the attending physician, being aware
that the patient had repeatedly tried to kill himself, or-
dered two attendants to watch him carefully. Two hours
after the patient had retired to bed, the physician, on
returning to pay him a visit, found him dead, strangled
by a strip from his shirt, rolled into a cord and tied
around his neck, notwithstanding that the two attendants had never left the room—at least they said so.‡

* Taylor: *op. cit.*, p. 440; Wharton and Stillé: *op. cit.*, vol. iii,
p. 363; Tidy: *op. cit.*, part ii, p. 443.

† " British and Foreign Med.-Chir. Rev.," 1852.

‡ "Ann. Med.-Psycholog.," t. iv, p. 113.

On the other hand, strangulation is often homicidal. In such cases the murderers either do too little or too much, in endeavoring to give the impression that death was suicidal, and so divert suspicion from themselves. Thus, in the well-known case of Sir Edmund Godfrey, who was strangled near Somerset House with a twisted handkerchief very forcibly applied, the sword of the deceased being afterward passed through his body, his gloves, etc., placed upon the bank so as to give the impression that death was due to suicide, the presence of a bruise extending around the neck, the fact of one of the cervical vertebræ being fractured, the lividity of the face, etc., proved that the deceased baronet had not committed suicide, but had been murdered.*

In another instance in which a person was strangled by a nurse in an infirmary, the latter, apparently from force of habit, laid the deceased out in her usual manner, smoothing the clothes under the body, placing the arms straight by the side, hands open, legs at full length, etc., entirely unconscious that such a condition of things was entirely inconsistent with the statement that death was suicidal, considering the amount of violence that must have been exerted in causing death.†

In the well-known case of Bartholomew Pourpre, the victim was first strangled and then suspended from a tree. The blood found in the mouth of the deceased, and the fact that the teeth were knocked in, proved conclusively that violence had been committed, the murderer being probably the father.‡

* Compare Beck: *op. cit.*, vol. ii, p. 206; Guy and Ferrier: *op. cit.*, 295.

† Taylor: *op. cit.*, p. 442.   ‡ Beck: *op. cit.*, vol. ii, p. 191.

Strangulation is sometimes produced accidentally. Cases have occurred, for example, where death was due to compression of the windpipe by straps or strings habitually worn around the necks of persons engaged in carrying heavy baskets of fish or vegetables for sale. Thus, a young woman who was employed to carry fish in a basket on her back, by means of a strap passing around her neck and shoulders, was found dead sitting on a stone wall, the trachea being compressed by the strap, which had been raised through the slipping off of the basket. In such cases, if trustworthy and disinterested witnesses testify that the body was found apparently in the position it occupied at the time of death, and in the absence of any evidence of criminal violence having been committed, there need be but little hesitation in attributing death to accidental suicide.

Death from Suffocation by Hanging.—In this mode of death the body is suspended by the neck, the weight of the body acting as the compressing force. If the neck is compressed beneath the thyroid cartilage, death is usually due to asphyxia, and is rapid; but if just beneath the chin, as is usually the case in executions, it is due to congestion of the brain (apoplexy), and is slow. In most cases death is due rather to the effects of both causes combined. Occasionally, death is caused immediately by pressure upon the spinal cord through fracture or displacement of the odontoid process of the second cervical vertebra. The hyoid bone and thyroid cartilage have also in some instances been fractured.* Death from fracture of the vertebræ in hanging, however, is not so frequent as is usually supposed. The post-mortem appearances

* Casper: *op. cit.*, vol. ii, p. 174.

observed in cases of death from hanging do not differ essentially from those already described in death from strangulation. Indeed, the mere inspection of the body will not enable the examiner to state positively that death was due to hanging. The flow of saliva out of the mouth, down the chin, and straight down the chest, is possibly one of the most positive signs of this kind of death; but the absence of such a flow would hardly justify the examiner in stating that death was not due to hanging. It is also extremely difficult to determine, when a body is found dead from hanging, whether the death should be regarded as accidental, suicidal, or homicidal.

Death from hanging is undoubtedly often due to accident, especially in children, who frequently play at hanging, with fatal results. On the other hand, in adults death by hanging is usually suicidal. From the fact that very young children rarely commit suicide, it might be supposed that the age of the deceased might assist the examiner to some extent in determining the cause of death by hanging. It must be remembered, though, that suicide has been committed by hanging by a boy of nine, and it may be added in this connection, by a man of ninety-seven years of age.

Death by hanging is, nevertheless, in some cases homicidal. Thus, in the case of a man named Hebner, who was found dead hanging in the garret with his hands tied behind his back and his handkerchief drawn over his face, it was shown that the rope had been tied around his neck in a "sailor's knot," which fact led to the conviction and execution of his murderers—a sailor, Ludlam, and a Mrs. Hughes, who kept the house in which the murder was committed.*

Death from Suffocation by Drowning.—In death from drowning, suffocation is caused by the presence of some liquid, usually water, which, interfering with the passage of air into the respiratory passages, acts even more effectually than when the throat is compressed externally, as in strangulation or hanging—the water entering even the bronchial tubes and air-vesicles. A human being, as a general rule, dies if submerged for a period of from four to five minutes. In order that a person should be suffocated by drowning, it is not necessary, however, that the whole body should be submerged. It is of no uncommon occurrence to find the dead bodies of persons, such as drunkards and epileptics, lying face downward in shallow pools into which they had fallen and by which they had been suffocated. The external signs presented by a drowned person will vary with the length of time the body has been in the water. Supposing the body not to have been in the water longer than two or three hours, and not to have been inspected immediately after removal, the face will be found pale, the eyes half open, the eyelids livid, the pupils dilated, the mouth usually open, the tongue swollen, often indented by the teeth, the lips and nostrils covered with a mucous froth. The skin usually presents the condition known as *goose-flesh*, and the penis is retracted. In addition, abrasions are often found upon the body, especially upon the hands, which frequently contain particles of sand, gravel, mud, and pieces of wood grasped by the drowning person in his struggle for life. Internally, the lungs are

* Beck: *op. cit.*, vol. II, p. 190.

found distended, overlapping the heart, sodden and doughy, owing to the water drawn in, and full of bloody mucous froth. In cases in which the lungs contain little or no water, the water will be found in the pleural cavities, into which it has transuded. Frequently, water is found in the stomach, together with parts of weeds, sand, and mud, such as are present in the pond or river in which the person was drowned. As a general rule, the right side of the heart only is gorged with dark blood, though both sides of the heart may be so distended.

The remaining organs do not present any characteristic changes. As the human body is somewhat heavier than water, the body of a drowned person will remain submerged until, through the development of putrefying gases, it becomes sufficiently light to float. The time elapsing between the moment when a person is drowned and that at which the body will come to the surface varies with the temperature of the air and water, the buoyancy of the latter, the age, sex, the constitution of the individual. In summer a body may float within twenty-four hours after drowning. A drowned body will rise to the surface sooner in salt than in fresh water. Fat bodies float sooner than thin bodies, and the bodies of women float sooner than those of men. Though a matter of importance, it is often impossible to state positively, in the case of a body floating in the water, supposed to have been drowned, the length of time that has elapsed since life became extinct. In this connection it can only be stated that the mucous froth and water usually found in the lungs of drowned persons disappear after putrefaction sets in; or when the body has been exposed for any great length of time to the air.

Death from drowning is usually accidental or suicidal—
rarely homicidal, except, however, in the case of infants,
which are frequently gotten rid of in this way.   But it
must be borne in mind that a person might be murdered
and then thrown into a river or pond with the idea that
death would be attributed to drowning.   Therefore, the
body of a drowned person should be always most carefully examined for marks of violence.   On the other hand,
the presence of wounds upon a body found dead floating
in the water would not prove that the case was one of
homicide, since suicides have frequently inflicted wounds
upon themselves before drowning.   Even the fact that the
limbs are found tied together, or that a stone or a heavy
weight is suspended from the neck of a body taken out
of the water, would not necessarily indicate homicide,
as suicide has often been committed in that manner.

Resuscitation.—While the best method of resuscitation
of a drowned person is not strictly a medico-legal question,
as the propriety of the treatment of drowned persons
has been severely criticized at coroners' inquests, a few
words in connection with this subject may not seem
inappropriate..   In attempting to resuscitate a drowned
person, the first thing to do is to remove all clothing
from the neck and chest.   The body should then be wiped
dry, and covered with dry clothes.   The mucous froth
that has collected within the nostrils, mouth, and throat
must be cleaned out, the tongue pulled forward, and
kept from falling back and in this way covering the larynx.
The body should then be placed at full length, face
downward, with the forehead resting on one arm, so as
to allow all fluids to run out of the mouth.   Ammonia,
snuff, aromatic vinegar, may now be cautiously applied

to the nostrils. If by these means respiration has not
been restored, the body must be placed upon its back,
and the head slightly raised. The arms should be gently
carried outward and upward, raised above the head,

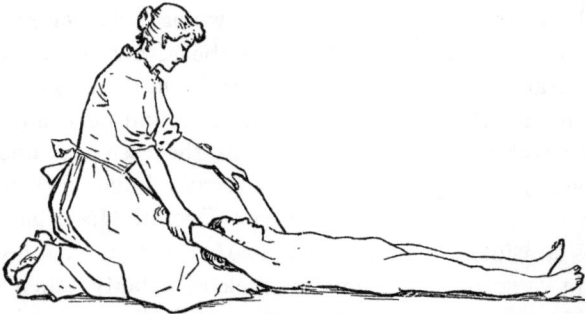

Fig. 24.—Resuscitation after drowning: first movement.

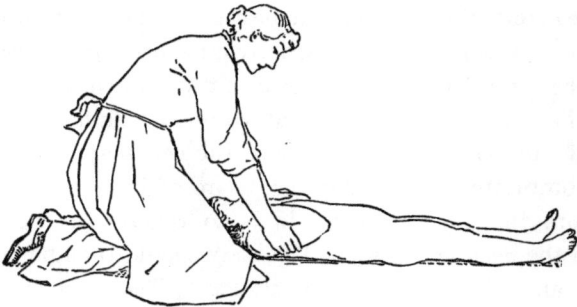

Fig. 25.—Resuscitation after drowning: second movement.

and kept momentarily in that position (Fig. 24). By
these movements, which should take about two seconds,
inspiration is effected and the air passes into the chest. The
arms should then be lowered and brought closely to the
sides of the chest, the lower part of the breast-bone being

at the same time compressed (Fig. 25). These movements, by which expiration is effected and air driven out of the chest, should also be made in about two seconds. These alternate movements of the arms should be repeated at this rate—that is, fifteen times a minute—until spontaneous breathing commences. Heat may then be applied either in the form of a warm bath or friction. When the power of swallowing returns, a little warm brandy and water may be given, and then the patient should be put to bed and allowed to sleep. This treatment should be persisted in for several hours, except in those cases where the body has been long under water and is taken out cold and rigid—where there is complete insensibility, no spontaneous breathing, entire absence of the heart-beat, the eyelids half closed, the lower jaw stiff, the mucous froth continually escaping from the nostrils and mouth. On the other hand, slight flushing and convulsive twitches of the face, returning warmth of the skin, gasping and sobbing, breathing movements of the body and limbs, are signs indicating speedy recovery.

CHAPTER VIII.

Rape upon Children—Rape upon Adults—Rape upon the Dead—
Rape by Females—Unnatural Crimes.

RAPE, medico-legally, is the carnal knowledge of a
woman forcibly and against her will.* At one time the
punishment for rape was death, castration, fine, or imprisonment. At the present day rape is regarded, in this
country at least, as a felony, and is punished by fine
and imprisonment for a term of years. From the fact
that, as a general rule, the crime of rape is committed
in the absence of witnesses, the law usually admits the
testimony of the victim to substantiate the charge.
It is very essential that medical testimony should be
obtained as corroborative evidence, as probably nine-
tenths of the accusations of rape are false. While it is
true, as just mentioned, that rape is a crime usually
attempted without witnesses, cases have occurred in
which a woman has been ravished, one criminal aiding
the other as he accomplished his purpose by forcibly
overcoming the resistance offered by the victim. Thus,
in one instance reported, one man held the woman down
on a bed by the neck, thus enabling the other to accomplish
his purpose. In another case the head of the victim
was firmly held by the accomplice of the ravisher between
his thighs.† In another revolting case an idiot girl was

* Guy and Ferrier: *op. cit.*, p. 59; Tidy: *op. cit.*, part II, p. 186.
† Taylor: *op. cit.*, sixth edition, p. 708.

ravished successively by two men, each man aiding in turn the other in holding the girl.* At one time, in cases of rape, the law demanded proofs of penetration as well as emission on the part of the male. At present, proof is only required of vulval penetration, without the hymen being necessarily ruptured.

Rape of young children, as might be expected, is far commoner than that of adult women, children being incapable of offering much resistance, even when old enough to realize the nature and consequences of the act. Indeed, of one hundred and thirty-six individuals examined by Casper † upon whom rape had been committed, ninety-nine, or nearly 73 per cent., were little children under twelve years of age. Owing, however, to the superstition prevailing in Europe, among the lower classes, that an old gonorrhœa is cured by intercourse with a virgin, rape of young children is far more common abroad than in America. Thus, among the lower orders in Ireland, a delusion prevails that a man can get rid of an obstinate clap that has "foiled the doctors," by having sexual intercourse with a virgin, and therefore a young child is selected as the easiest mode of accomplishing the purpose.‡

In cases of the insane, idiotic, or only feeble-minded, or if the victim be under sixteen years of age, the consent of the female will not be accepted as an excuse for the act. Difficulty, however, is sometimes experienced in determining to what extent the reason of the female alleged to have been overcome is affected. It may be mentioned, in this connection, that the fact that a woman

---

* Casper: *op. cit.*, vol. III, p. 283.　　　　† *Op. cit.*, p. 307.
‡ Wilde: " Medical Times and Gazette," September 10, 1853,

in a state of stupor has been subjected to rape would not be an excuse for the act; neither would submission from fear or from ignorance of the nature of the crime. Further, even if the character of the woman was notoriously bad, yet, if it was in evidence that such a woman, a prostitute, for example, had been forced against her will, the act would be a rape. Under such circumstances, it must be admitted that on account of the bad character of the woman the evidence would have to be very strong to convict. Nevertheless, in the Bates case, which occurred some years ago in Boston, four men were convicted on the evidence of an eye-witness and sentenced to five years' imprisonment for having successively violated a strumpet without and against her consent.*

In every alleged case of rape it is most important that the medical examiner should note exactly the time of making his examination, and also determine, so far as possible, the time elapsing since the act was committed, as this may subsequently become important evidence in proving whether or not the child or woman entered complaint at once, and submitted without delay to an examination, as also in enabling the defendant to prove an alibi. The female should be visited by the medical examiner as soon as possible after the perpetration of the crime, as all traces of rape, if such has been committed, may disappear in a few days; or, in the event of the accusation being a false one, the woman should not be allowed time to produce artificially evidences simulating those of rape. In alleged cases of rape, a medical examination is not compulsory; but if a woman under such circumstances refuses to have an examination made, that in itself would

* Wharton and Stillé: *op. cit.*, p. 182.

be strong presumptive evidence against the truth of the charge.

In cases of rape the medical examiner may expect to find marks of violence about the genitalia, wounds, bruises, etc., on both the person of the woman and of the accused, spermatic stains and blood-stains on the person and clothing of both, gonorrhœa or syphilis in one or both. Rape perpetrated upon young children by men is attended, as might be expected, on account of the great disproportion in size of the sexual organs, with far more severe local injuries than when committed upon adult women. Indeed, the absence of any such marks of violence would be strong proof of the charge of rape made being a false one.

If a child be examined within two or three days after the commission of the crime, the vulva will be usually found inflamed and swollen, and more or less covered with clotted blood, which has oozed from the abraded mucous membrane. From the vagina there flows a muco-purulent, ropy discharge of a yellowish-green color, which stains and stiffens the linen. Urination is frequently painful, from the inflammation extending to the urethra. The hymen may be only lacerated or entirely effaced. Indeed, it has been stated upon the highest authority * that in 999 cases out of 1000 where defloration has taken place, the hymen is destroyed, and this is probably true, at least so far as regards girls arrived at the age of puberty and upward.

Too much importance, however, must not be attached by the medical examiner to the presence or absence of the hymen as disproving or proving a rape. Indeed, as a matter of fact, in most cases of rape upon young children,

* Devergié: *op. cit.*, p. 346.

the hymen escapes injury entirely, probably because it is situated in such cases far back. On the other hand, the hymen may have been destroyed, not necessarily by rape, but by disease, accident, as in the case of a young girl who fell from a tree upon a sharp stake which, penetrating the vagina, destroyed the hymen,* or even intentionally, the object being in the latter case to extort money by a false accusation of rape.

It may be mentioned in this connection that the hymen, when once destroyed, is never renewed, the vagina and external parts recovering, however, in time their healthy tonicity.

The vagina is frequently found very much dilated in the case of young children who have been assaulted. The medical examiner should bear in mind that such a dilated condition of the vagina has often been artificially produced by the introduction of hard bodies with the view of fitting the children for sexual intercourse. Thus, in a revolting case mentioned by Casper,† a woman, with the above object, dilated the vagina of her child, a girl of only ten years of age, first with two and then with four fingers, finally stuffing it with a long stone.

It is very important that the muco-purulent discharge from the vagina just referred to as following rape should not be confounded with either infantile leucorrhœa (vaginitis), gangrenous inflammation of the vulva, or gonorrhœa. Infantile leucorrhœa occurs in unhealthy, particularly strumous children, whose hygienic surroundings are of the worst character. It should be borne in mind by the medical examiner that the presence of such a discharge

* Wharton and Stillé: *op. cit.*, vol. III, p. 201.
† Casper: *op. cit.*, vol. III, p. 318.

in a young child is often taken advantage of by an unscrupulous mother to bring a charge of assault against an innocent man. Gangrenous inflammation of the vulva, less common than infantile leucorrhœa, is found among neglected children suffering from inanition, exhaustion, etc. As a general rule, the absence of blood and of bruises in a young child alleged to have been assaulted would be strong proof that the vaginal discharge was due rather to leucorrhœa or gangrenous inflammation than to the effects of violence.

In endeavoring to determine whether a vaginal discharge be due to gonorrhœa rather than to violence, the medical examiner should bear in mind that a gonorrhœal discharge does not make its appearance until between the fourth and the eighth day, and is usually much more profuse and lasts longer than the muco-purulent discharge incidental to rape. In all alleged cases of rape it is important to determine whether the accused be affected with gonorrhœa or syphilis, since if the child be so diseased there would be strong proof of the guilt of the accused. It is possible, however, that either gonorrhœa or syphilis might be communicated to young children either accidentally or intentionally by means of sponges and towels that had been previously used by persons affected with these diseases, and that advantage may be taken of this to accuse an innocent man of felonious assault. Thus, according to Dr. Ryan, two children were accidentally infected with gonorrhœa by using the sponge of a servant girl who had the disease.* In another case reported by Hamilton, syphilis was communicated to a girl of only six years of age by a boy of nineteen, the infectious matter

* "London Medical Gazette," vol. LXVII, p. 744.

having been communicated by the fingers.* On the other hand, a tradesman of irreproachable character was accused of having violated a girl of eleven years of age, and of having communicated to her the gonorrhœa. It was shown, however, that the accused was free from the disease, and subsequently that the child had been purposely infected by the paramour of the mother, who knew that he had the disease at that time, the mother, having failed to extort money from the tradesman, taking

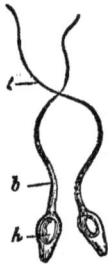

Fig. 26.—Spermatozoa of man : *h*, Apparent nucleus ; *b*, body ; *t*, tail.

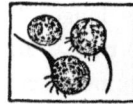

Fig. 27. — Trichomonas vaginalis, showing the large heads, with granules and cilia.

this means of frightening him to comply with her request.†

In all cases of alleged rape, the clothing and person of the female and of the accused should be carefully examined for seminal stains, which stiffen the linen or other wearing apparel very much as gum or albumin will do. There are several methods by which seminal stains can be identified, such as the yellow color assumed when gently heated or when dissolved in weak nitric acid, or by the odor when moistened with warm water.

* " Dublin Medical Press," vol. xx, No. 511, 1848.

† Casper: *op. cit.*, vol. iii, p. 301.

The only positive proof of semen, however, is the presence of spermatozoa, as shown by the microscope. A convenient method of obtaining the spermatozoa for microscopic examination is to cut out a piece of the material stained with the seminal discharge and place it in a watch-glass containing distilled water. After the material has been thoroughly soaked, a drop of the liquid should then be transferred to a glass slide, and the latter placed on the stage of the microscope. In case of examining the hair of the female, to which the spermatozoa cling with great tenacity, the hair should be moistened with a drop of weak ammonia and examined with the microscope after the liquid has evaporated. The spermatozoa (Fig. 26) present a very characteristic appearance when viewed with the microscope, though resembling somewhat the flagellate infusoria, for which they were mistaken when first discovered. A spermatozoon consists of an ovoidal head, which tapers into a filamentary appendage or tail, about ten times as long as the head, and which, when the spermatozoon is alive, vibrates with astonishing rapidity. The spermatozoa vary in number and size, measuring on an average between $\frac{1}{500}$ and $\frac{1}{600}$ of an inch, and may be sometimes found still living and quite active even a week after sexual intercourse. The movements of the spermatozoa are arrested by water and cold, retarded by acids, and stimulated by alkalies. The spermatozoa retain individual life long after the death of the body, having been seen moving about as long as from eighty to one hundred hours after death.* In the dried condition the spermatozoa may be identified years after death.

* Taylor: *op. cit.*, p. 693.

Spermatozoa are found in the semen of man from the age of puberty to a very advanced period of life—ninety years and upward. Spermatozoa are often absent, however, in the semen; for example, in that of young men addicted to excessive venery or suffering from debilitating diseases. The absence of spermatozoa from stains cannot, then, be regarded as proof that such stains are not seminal in origin. In old seminal stains, as the spermatozoa are frequently found in fragments, the medical examiner should be extremely cautious under such circumstances in not mistaking for them the fibers of organic bodies that might accidentally be present. The only living animalcule that might be mistaken for a spermatozoon is the *trichomonas vaginalis* (Fig. 27) occasionally found in the vaginal mucus of uncleanly females. The trichomonas vaginalis is, however, readily distinguished from a spermatozoon, in that its head is much larger, granular, and armed with a row of from four to six cilia. In connection with the subject of the rape of children, it should be mentioned that death not infrequently results from mortification or peritonitis brought on by violent laceration of the vagina or perineum.

Rape upon Adult Women.—In cases of alleged rape upon adult women, the medical examiner may be questioned as to the possibility of a healthy, vigorous adult woman being overcome by one man. No positive answer should be given to so general a question, as all such cases must be judged according to particular circumstances. The relative size of the man and woman, whether the woman's life had been threatened, her condition at the time, whether she was in full possession of her faculties or stupefied by drink, whether narcotized, hypnotized, or under the influence of anæsthetics, must all be taken into careful consideration before the examiner commits himself to the expression of a positive opinion. However different the views of medical jurists may be in regard to the possibility of an adult woman being raped, the question, as a matter of fact, has been settled *in foro* in the affirmative. Thus, in a well-known case where a young woman twenty years of age, unmarried, and of excellent character, confessed to her mother immediately on her return home that she had been violated in a pathway near by, in spite of having offered every resistance in her power, by a soldier twenty-two years of age, who had accidentally met her, the accused was convicted and sentenced to five years' imprisonment.* In another instance in which a young woman twenty-five years of age, strong and healthy, was induced by a man to go into the Thiergarten in Berlin, in the dark, all the evidence went to show that she was raped, notwithstanding the vigorous resistance offered. The defendant was convicted and condemned to four years' penal servitude.†

The question has often been asked of the medical expert whether a woman could be raped while asleep. The Medical Faculty of Leipsic decided that question in the affirmative in 1669; "dormientem in sella virginem insciam deflorari posse." Notwithstanding, it seems incredible that a woman could sleep so soundly as to be unconscious of having sexual intercourse. Such, indeed, was the opinion of Valentin, who, in commenting upon the above

---

* Henke: "Zeits. Erg.," Heft 41, pp. 21–44.
† Casper: *op. cit.*, vol. iii, p. 311.

decision, shrewdly observes: "Non omnes dormiunt qui clausos et conniventes habent oculos."*

It should be mentioned, in this connection, that excitable, emotional women, under the influence of ether and chloroform, especially if the period be that of their menses, are very apt to imagine that they are having sexual intercourse with their husbands, lovers, or even with the surgeon or dentist who may be operating upon them. So true is this that it is of the utmost importance for surgeons and dentists to insist upon the presence of witnesses during the performance of operations upon women under the influence of anæsthetics. Indeed, in the absence of witnesses under such circumstances, professional men have been charged and convicted of rape, though without doubt entirely innocent of the crime, and, extraordinary as it may appear, even though the women were never at any time examined medically.† Unfortunately, in the case of alleged rape upon adult women, the medical examination usually made is postponed so long that even if the crime has been committed all traces of it have disappeared. If the woman has offered much resistance, bruises will usually be found upon the thighs and legs, and sometimes also upon the arms and trunk. The most important proofs of rape upon adult women are, however, derived from the condition of the sexual organs and the hymen, and the presence of blood and semen. Among such proofs may be mentioned the soreness, swelling, laceration of the vulva and vagina, rupture of the hymen, the presence of blood and semen upon the persons and clothes of the woman and man.

* Valentini, Michaelis Bernhardi: "Novellæ Medico-legales," Frankfort ad Moenum, 1711, Introd. Part ii, pp. 30, 31.

† "Philadelphia Medical Examiner," December, 1854, p. 705.

But it must be remembered that frequently women affected with leucorrhœa or vaginitis, in both of which diseases there is a discharge from the vagina simulating that produced by violence, take advantage of their condition to charge innocent men with having committed rape upon them. Further, while the discharge in leucorrhœa is mucous in character, that of intense vaginitis may be so purulent as to make it impossible to distinguish it from that of gonorrhœa. Under such circumstances, the fact that a man has gonorrhœa would not be proof that he had committed an assault upon the woman charging him with rape, since the purulent discharge in the woman might be due to vaginitis rather than to gonorrhœa acquired from the man.

In the case of alleged rape upon adult women, as upon children, much importance cannot be attached to the presence or absence of the hymen as disproving or proving a rape, for the reasons already given. If there be, however, other signs of violence, a ruptured or lacerated hymen would be strong corroborative evidence of a rape having been committed.

Proof of Rape in the Dead.—Occasionally the medical examiner may be called upon to determine whether a woman found dead had been violated before death. In the absence of witnesses, and in view of the fact that the prosecutrix can make no statement, the evidence will be necessarily entirely of a medical character. But in such cases, even if all the signs of sexual intercourse were present, it would be impossible for the medical examiner to state whether the woman had or had not given her consent. Again, on the supposition that the deceased woman had been violated and murdered, it might be impossible to state positively whether the murderer and ravisher were one and the same person. Indeed, a woman found dead and violated may have been murdered first and violated afterward, and not necessarily by the same person, for, horrible as the thought may be, violation of the dead is less rare than might be supposed. Indeed, it was of such common occurrence in ancient times that classical writers refer to the necessity of undertakers being watched to prevent them violating the bodies of deceased women committed to their charge.

In a remarkable case of modern times reported by Klose, a clergyman, while watching the supposed corpse of a young girl, gratified his lust upon her. Animation being, however, only temporarily suspended, the apparent corpse awakened and the woman became pregnant.* Was the clergyman the father? might naturally be asked.

In the case of a very young girl being found dead and violated, the probability is that the child had been ravished and then murdered, the ravisher hoping by that means to escape the consequences of his crime.

Rape by Females.—It would hardly be supposed that a rape could or would be committed by a female upon a male. As a matter of fact, nevertheless, such cases have occurred. Thus, in one instance a female of eighteen years of age compelled a boy fourteen years old to gratify her. In another, a girl of the same age ravished two male children, one thirteen, the other eleven years old, and gave them both syphilis, with which she was affected. In the last instance the girl appeared to be unable to gratify her desires with adults on account of the narrowness of her vagina.†

* Wharton and Stillé: *op. cit.*, vol. III, p. 184.
† Wharton and Stillé: *op. cit.*, vol. III, p. 207.

Casper relates a case in which a chaste, modest-looking nurse was in the habit of making a boy six years of age sleep with her, and in the attempt to gratify her desires in this way gave the child gonorrhœa.*

Unnatural Crimes.—Though not germane to the subject of this section, crimes against nature, committed either with man or beast, unnatural crimes, sodomy, pæderastia, tribadism, bestiality, may as appropriately be considered in their medico-legal relations here as elsewhere. While of frequent occurrence in the East, such practices are rare in America, and are criminal and punishable by imprisonment for a term of years. In cases of sodomy, both parties are held to be equally guilty, unless the person on whom the act was committed refused consent, or was a minor, an idiot, or feeble-minded. In recent cases laceration of the sphincter ani, bruises and fissures, and blood about the anus may be observed. Unless, however, the examination be made very soon after perpetration of the act, all traces will have disappeared. Characteristic appearances are presented by persons addicted to such practices. Among the most conspicuous may be mentioned a funnel-shaped condition of the anus, which is usually enlarged, smooth, and destitute of rugæ.†
Chancres and venereal warts are also not uncommonly present.

* Casper: *op. cit.*, vol. III, p. 283.
† "Multò magis frequentem tam nefandé coitûs usum significare poterit ipsius. Podicis constitutio, qui cùm ex Natura rugosus existat, ex hujus modi congressu laevis, ac planus efficitur, obliterantur enim rugæ illæ in ani curriculo existerites, ob assiduam membri attritionem" (Zacchias, Pauli: *a, Quaestionum Medico-legalium,* Lib. v, Tit. I, Quaest. I, p. 383; *b,* Lib. II, Tit. II, Quaest. II, p. 288).

CHAPTER IX.

Signs of Pregnancy—Uncertainty of Duration of Pregnancy—
Premature and Protracted Gestation—Precocious Pregnancy—
Unconscious Pregnancy—Pregnancy in the Dead—Corpus Lu-
teum.

THE subject of pregnancy is an important one medico-
legally, as women, on the one hand, frequently deny that
they are pregnant, in order to avoid disgrace or to procure
an abortion, and on the other hand as often affirm that
they are pregnant, having no reason to think that they are
in that condition, in order to extort money, to defraud the
heir-at-law, to avoid attendance upon a trial, to stay
capital punishment. A pregnant female was exempted
by the old Roman law from capital punishment,* and the
law is the same in most modern countries, hence the sum-
moning of twelve matrons or discreet women in old times,
under the writ of *de ventre inspiciendo*, to determine whether
a woman was pregnant or quick with child—an office now
performed by the city's physician or by a jury of physicians.

Actions for damages against physicians and others, involving questions of pregnancy, often arise in cases in which
it is claimed that errors in diagnosis were committed, or
that slanderous reports were circulated against the character of a virtuous woman.

The **signs of pregnancy** may be described as being of
two kinds: uncertain and certain, or positive. The former

* "Quod prægnatis mulieris damnatæ pœna differatur quoad
pariat" (Beck: *op. cit.*, vol. I, p. 250).

kind, as the name implies, is, from a medico-legal point of view at least, of but little importance as compared with the latter.

Uncertain Signs of Pregnancy.—Among these may be mentioned the suppression of the catamenia, morning sickness, enlargement of the abdomen, quickening, development of the breasts, kiesteine in the urine, the violet color of the vagina.

Suppression of the menses, when occurring only after intercourse, in a woman who had hitherto been regular, may be regarded as a very probable sign of pregnancy. As the menses may continue, however, throughout pregnancy,* may only appear during that condition,† or may never appear at all,‡ even in women who bear children, and as they are also absent in certain diseases, it is evident that neither their absence nor their presence can be regarded as a proof of pregnancy or non-pregnancy. But it should be mentioned that not infrequently women desiring to conceal their pregnancy stain their linen with blood and even with menstrual blood, borrowed for that purpose.

Nausea is usually an accompaniment of pregnancy, occurring frequently as early as the second or third week after conception. It generally passes away about the time of quickening, but may continue throughout the whole period of pregnancy. In many cases of pregnancy nausea is absent; on the other hand, it is of frequent occurrence in many diseases. But little importance can therefore be attached to nausea alone as a sign of pregnancy.

* "Lancet," February, 1856, p. 197.

† Wharton and Stillé: *op. cit.,* vol. III, p. 4.

‡ "Lancet," September, 1853, p. 206; Montgomery: "Signs of Pregnancy," second edition, p. 77.

The *enlargement of the abdomen* in a pregnant woman becomes evident at the end of the third month, the uterus then rising out of the pelvic cavity. By the end of the fifth month the uterus is half-way between the pelvis and the umbilicus, and at the sixth month at the umbilicus. During the seventh month it is at a point midway between the umbilicus and ensiform cartilage, reaching at the end of the eighth month the ensiform cartilage. During the last month the tumor widens and falls forward. Enlargement of the abdomen may be due, however, to ovarian dropsy and tumors, ascites, flatus of the intestines, impacted feces, enlargement of the spleen and kidney, and distention of the bladder. The medical examiner would certainly not be justified, therefore, in expressing the opinion that a woman was pregnant simply because there was enlargement of the abdomen.

The sad case of Lady Flora Hastings, who lost her position at court and died of a broken heart, the court physician having stated that she was pregnant on account of the enlargement of her abdomen, which was subsequently shown to be due to disease, may serve as a warning to those obstetricians who are so ready to swear on the flimsiest kind of evidence that a woman is pregnant.

Quickening is the first perception by the mother of the movements of the fœtus. These movements, which occur usually some time between the sixteenth and the twenty-fourth week, may be due either to the uterus or to the fœtus. Nervous, excitable women, especially those wanting children, frequently imagine, however, they are pregnant, attributing the movements of their intestines or contractions of their abdominal muscles, or symptoms due to disease, to a fœtus. Queen Mary of England, on the introduction of the Pope's legate, is said to have distinctly felt "the babe leap in her womb," though what she felt was not the child she longed for, her condition being due, not to pregnancy, but to dropsy. Quickening, being entirely a subjective symptom, is, therefore, a very unreliable sign of pregnancy.

The *breasts* usually develop during the period of pregnancy, becoming larger and fuller as the secretion of milk increases. Large veins make their appearance, the nipples become more prominent, the areola widens and darkens in hue, especially in brunettes. Enlargement of the breasts, however, is not a proof of pregnancy, inasmuch as it occurs in cases of uterine fibroids, and in various other ovarian and uterine disorders. Even the secretion of milk would not warrant the statement that a woman was pregnant, since milk is secreted occasionally by elderly women who have long since ceased to bear children, as also by young girls still unmarried and virgins. Thus, for example, in one well-known instance a woman sixty-eight years old, who had not borne a child for more than twenty years, nursed several grandchildren, one after the other. In another case, a servant girl, being disturbed at night by the cries of a child with whom she slept and whom it was desired to wean, put it to her breast merely to keep it quiet. In a short time, to her surprise, the breasts supplied the child with all the milk it wanted.* Indeed, there have even been cases in which the secretion of milk by men has been so copious that they have been able to perform the office of wet-nurse for years. Thus, among other cases may be mentioned that of a well-known colored man fifty-five years of age, who officiated for several years as wet-nurse

* Beck: *op. cit.*, vol. I, p. 267.

in the family of his mistress.   In the winter of 1849–50 an
athletic man twenty-two years of age was shown at the
clinic of the Jefferson Medical College, of Philadelphia,
whose left mamma had become greatly developed and which
secreted milk copiously.*

By *kiestcine* is understood the fatty pellicle which forms
on the urine of pregnant women that has been standing
some days.   It appears to consist of a combination of
casein and phosphates.   As kiesteine is not peculiar to the
urine of pregnant women, being found sometimes in the
urine of men, its presence cannot be regarded as a proof
of pregnancy.

Jacquemin's Test: The violet color of the vagina, appearing about the fourth week of gestation, due to venous congestion, may be regarded as a valuable sign of pregnancy,
but an uncertain one, since it is not invariably present.

Certain Signs of Pregnancy.—Among the so-called certain
or positive signs of pregnancy are included ballottement,
change in the form of the body and cervix of the uterus,
the active movements of the child, the uterine and umbilical sounds, the pulsation of the fœtal heart.

Ballottement: By ballottement is determined the presence of a fœtus about the fifth or sixth month of pregnancy.
In performing it, the woman is made to stand upright and
the finger of one hand is introduced into the vagina up to
the body of the uterus, while the other hand is placed upon
the abdomen, so as to steady the uterine tumor.   If the
tip of the finger be now suddenly pushed up against the
uterus, a sensation, should a fœtus be present, will be felt
like that of a body rising and falling in a liquid.   While

* Dunglison: "Human Physiology," eighth edition, vol. ii, p.
520.

ballottement is regarded by most obstetricians as a most reliable method of determining the presence of a fœtus, it should always be borne in mind, in applying it, that any floating tumor in the uterus will impart the same sensation to the finger as that due to a fœtus, and that the possibility of such a tumor being present, though the occurrence is rare, should always be taken into consideration in deciding whether a woman is or is not pregnant.

Changes in the Form of the Body and Cervix of the Uterus: At about the fifth month of pregnancy the os uteri is directed backward, and has a velvet-like feel; the shortening of the cervix becomes evident shortly after this time and continues until the ninth month, when the cervix ceases to be distinguishable from the body of the uterus (Figs. 28, 29, 30). It must be admitted, however, that the shortening of the cervix, as a proof of pregnancy, cannot be greatly depended upon, as according to some obstetricians it does not occur during pregnancy, or, if at all, not until the last few days.*

The *active movements of the child* can usually be felt about the fifth month of pregnancy, or even earlier, by placing a cold hand upon the surface of the abdomen. Intestinal movements must not be mistaken, however, for those of a fœtus. It should be remembered, also, that not infrequently in cases of pregnancy the movements of the fœtus are not perceptible.

The *uterine sound,* a peculiar blowing or whistling sound, synchronous with the maternal pulse, and due probably to the passage of blood through the uterine arteries and placental vessels, can usually be heard over most of the

* " Edinburgh Medical Journal," March, 1859, p. 773; "American Medical Times," June 21, 1862.

abdomen as early as the middle of the third month of pregnancy, but more distinctly as pregnancy advances. As uterine sounds can, however, be heard in cases of enlargement of the uterus, as from tumors, such signs are very unreliable signs of pregnancy, and the same may be said

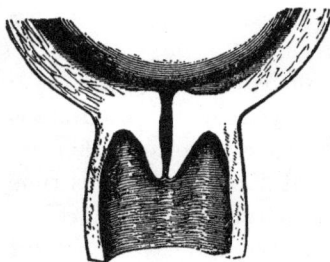

Fig. 28.—Cervix uteri (at about the fifth month of gestation), showing little or no absorption.

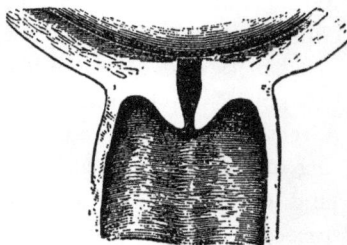

Fig. 29.—Cervix uteri (at about the sixth month of gestation), showing evident absorption.

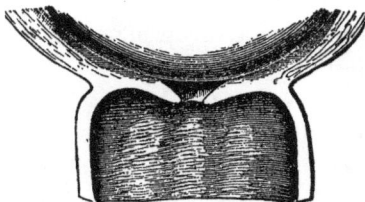

Fig. 30.—Cervix uteri at close of gestation, completely obliterated.

of the umbilical sounds due to the flow of blood through the umbilical vessels.

Pulsation of the Fœtal Heart: Indeed, of all the so-called "certain signs" of pregnancy, the pulsation of the fœtal heart is the only certain and positive one, and then only when it can be so distinctly heard as to be counted. The fœtal sound is not synchronous with the pulse of the mother, the fœtal heart beating at a rate of one hundred and thirty-six beats to the minute, and even faster. It resembles the ticking of a watch, and is heard over different parts of the abdomen, but best between the ilium and the umbilicus on either side. It may be heard as early as the middle of the fifth month, but much more distinctly as pregnancy advances.*

Responsibility of Mistaken Diagnosis.—As the so-called "certain signs" of pregnancy, with the exception of the pulsation of the fœtal heart, are only relatively more certain than the uncertain signs, the medical examiner should be extremely cautious, under any circumstances, in stating positively that a woman is pregnant, and especially if she be unmarried and of previously good character. On more than one occasion has the reputation of a virtuous woman been ruined and the happiness of her family destroyed by a too confident examiner mistaking a condition of disease for that of pregnancy. When once the virtue of an innocent woman has been thus impugned, and her previously good character taken away, though in time the injustice of the charge will surely be proved, reparation will come too late, and no atonement can be made for the wrong done the woman or the misery inflicted upon her family. Apart from the injury to the woman due to a mistake in diagnosis under such circumstances, the examiner should remember, even in the absence of any higher motive, that his own reputation as a medical expert may be at stake.

Cases of supposed pregnancy differ in one respect from other cases demanding the attention of the medical jurist —namely, there is no necessity that a positive opinion

* Scanzoni: "Lehrbuch der Geburtshülfe," vierte Auflage, Wien, 1867, Bd. i, S. 160.

should be expressed upon the subject. No harm can result from the medical examiner refusing to state positively whether a woman is pregnant or not. It is far better to give the woman, if unmarried and of good character, the benefit of the doubt, than positively commit yourself to the expression of an erroneous opinion in the case. It should always be remembered that nature will soon answer so positively the question whether a woman is or is not pregnant, that there will be no necessity of the examiner weighing the relative value of the uncertain and certain signs of pregnancy.

In cases of suspected pregnancy, where the best of all tests—that of time—cannot be waited for, and the exigencies of the case demand some expression of opinion, the medical examiner should never rely on a single symptom, but base his opinion upon the presence or absence of several of those signs of pregnancy just mentioned. In regard to supposed pregnancies in the early months of gestation, if any opinion at all is expressed it should be a most guarded one. Finally, in all cases of supposed pregnancy of any great importance, if there be any doubt in the mind of the medical examiner about any point, he should insist upon a consultation with another physician to share the responsibility.

Duration of Pregnancy.—The determination of the duration of pregnancy under certain circumstances, as in cases involving questions of legitimacy and inheritance, may become a matter, medico-legally, of the greatest importance. It should be stated, therefore, that the common idea of pregnancy lasting nine calendar months—273 to 276 days—is an incorrect one, since normal gestation lasts at least ten lunar months, or 280 days, the physiological presumption being that parturition occurs at the period which would correspond to the tenth menstrual period since the last one. The greatest difference of opinion prevails, however, as to what shall constitute the longest and shortest possible periods of gestation. The difference of opinion in this respect depends to a great extent upon our ignorance as to the exact moment of conception. As conception may take place at any moment of the period intervening between the menses, it is evident that there may be a difference on this account alone of twenty-eight days in the period of gestation, according as conception was supposed to have taken place immediately after the last menses, or before the period at which the menses would have occurred had not conception taken place.

Premature and Protracted Gestation.—Even, however, when this source of error is taken into account, the duration of pregnancy varies very much in different women on account of personal idiosyncrasies, as well as on account of other causes not understood. Obstetricians have claimed that mature children have been born as early as from 210 to 217 days,* and as late as from 313 even to 325 days † after sexual intercourse, there being a difference between these very exceptional extremes of as much as 96 days. Cases are not rare, however, in which the difference in the duration of gestation in cases of mature children amounts to as much as 44 days, the two extremes of gestation being 249 and 293 days respectively. It should be mentioned in this connection that while a child born after a period of protracted gestation is neither larger nor better developed than one born after the average period, a child

---

* Beck: *op. cit.*, vol. I, p. 599.
† Tidy: *op. cit.*, part II, pp. 68, 69.

born only seven months after sexual intercourse is always immature and imperfect—readily distinguishable from one born after the average period.* It is for this reason that the statement that a mature child is born seven months after sexual intercourse must be regarded as most exceptional.

Precocious Pregnancy.—In tropical countries women become pregnant at a much earlier age than in temperate climes. Thus, in India and Abyssinia it is no uncommon occurrence for girls of only eleven and twelve years of age to bear children. Pregnancy has been known to occur, however, even in children of only eight and nine years of age. Thus, it was reported † some years ago that a girl became pregnant at eight years and ten months of age and was delivered in due time of a child weighing seven pounds.

Late Pregnancy.—On the other hand, it is well known that women from sixty-three to seventy years of age have borne children.‡ Indeed, in one case it was reported that a woman at sixty-two years of age was delivered of triplets, the authenticity of which might well be doubted were it not for the high esteem in which the journal is held in which the statement appeared.§

Unconscious Pregnancy.—Under certain circumstances it may become a question whether a woman can become pregnant while unconscious. There can be no doubt of the possibility of such an occurrence, as it is well known that women have borne children in consequence of having

* Montgomery: "Signs and Symptoms of Pregnancy," second edition, London, 1856, pp. 523, 546.

† "Lancet," April 9, 1881, p. 601.

‡ Briand: "Manuel Complété de Méd. Legale," p. 137; "British Medical Journal," November 16, 1872, p. 570.

§ "Lancet," 1867, I, p. 727.

PLATE 2.

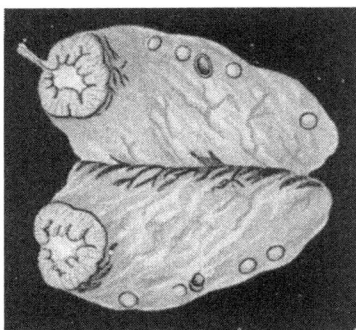

FIG. 2.—Ovary of woman at term of pregnancy, showing corpus luteum with firm white central clot.

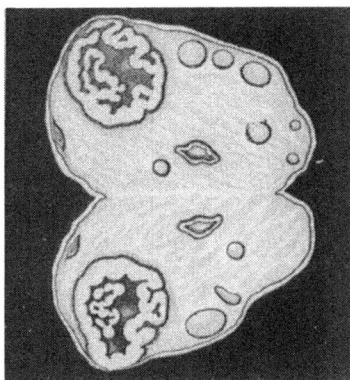

FIG. 1.—Ovary of woman twenty days after menstruation; besides large fresh corpus luteum are seen two smaller old ones, and Graafian follicles of different sizes (DALTON).

been ravished when in a state of unconsciousness induced by disease or by the use of narcotics or anæsthetics.*

Pregnancy in the Dead.—It not infrequently occurs that the medical examiner is required to determine whether a woman was pregnant at the time of her death, as, for example, in cases where the charge is that of seduction and murder. In considering the subject of putrefaction, it will be remembered that attention was called to the remarkable fact that the unimpregnated uterus will resist decomposition longer than any other organ in the body, and which makes it possible for the medical examiner to state positively, in some cases at least, even months after burial, whether a woman died pregnant or not. Further, even after years of interment, if the woman died pregnant and the fœtus had reached the period of ossification, traces of its bones will be found among those of its mother.

Corpus Luteum.—Importance was attached at one time to the presence or absence of a corpus luteum (Plate 2, Fig. 1), or the yellow body developed through modification of the lining membrane and coagulated blood of the Graafian follicle from which an ovum had escaped, as proving or disproving pregnancy. The author, however, like others,† has not infrequently found a fœtus in the uterus where there was no trace of a corpus luteum in either ovary; and, on the other hand, a well-developed corpus luteum, indistinguishable from that of pregnancy (Plate 2, Fig. 2), in the ovary of a married woman who had never been pregnant, and even in that of a virgin. The presence or absence of a corpus luteum cannot, then, be regarded as having any importance in medico-legal cases involving questions of pregnancy.

* Casper: *op. cit.*, vol. III, p. 307; "Philadelphia Examiner," December, 1854.   † Tidy: *op. cit.*, part II, p. 125.

CHAPTER X.

THE **procreative power** in the male begins at the age of
puberty, between fourteen and fifteen years of age, with
the full development of the testicles, the power of fecunda-
tion depending upon the presence of active spermatozoa
in the semen. The procreative power may continue to an
advanced period of life, spermatozoa being found, as already
mentioned, in the semen of very old men.

The procreative power begins in the female, as well
known, earlier than in the male—at about twelve to
thirteen years of age, and even earlier in tropical countries.

Impotence, or the inability for sexual intercourse, may
be due to masturbation, to the opium and the alcohol
habits, diseases of the nervous system, blows upon the head
and back, absence, deficiency, or malformation of the penis,
as hypospadias, epispadias, fistula in perineo. It should
be mentioned that there may be impotency without sterility
(absence of spermatozoa), as in those cases in which sexual
intercourse is prevented by malformation of the penis; and,
on the other hand, sterility without impotency, as in cases
of castration.

In connection with the absence of the testicles it should

154

be mentioned that their mere absence from the scrotum does not involve sterility, since such a condition may be simply due, as in crypsorchides, to the testicles not having descended into the scrotum from the inguinal canal, the semen, nevertheless, containing spermatozoa,* as is the case in the elephant and some other mammals which are normally crypsorchides. It may also be mentioned that the sterility of old men, in some cases at least, appears to be due to the sluggishness of their spermatozoa rather than to their absence from the semen.

Sterility, or the inability to conceive and to procreate their kind, in the female may be due to debility, leucor-rhœa, dysmenorrhœa, amenorrhœa, menorrhagia, absence or disease of the uterus or ovaries, imperforate vagina or hymen, occlusion of the uterus, etc. It is an interesting fact that while a woman may be sterile with one man, she may be fertile with another, it frequently happening that a woman, married for years without issue, in con-tracting a second marriage may bear children. In the female, as in the male, sterility (absence of ova) may exist without incapacity for sexual intercourse, and *vice versâ*.

Grounds for Divorce.—Impotence or sterility may constitute grounds for divorce proceedings on the part of husband or wife, provided it can be proved that the incapacity for sexual intercourse existed at or before the time of marriage. If such incapacity supervened, however, after marriage, as due to disease, there would be no grounds for such proceedings. In such cases a medical examination would, of course, be necessary, and while such an examination could not be made compulsory,

* Casper: *op. cit.*, vol. III, p. 256.

any refusal on the part of either of the contending parties
to submit to the same would certainly be injurious to
the cause of the party so refusing.

So-called "frigidity of constitution," or unwillingness
to submit to sexual intercourse, would not constitute
grounds for legal divorce, absolute proof being required
of incapacity for sexual intercourse, or of severe and
intense pain being suffered by indulging in it, as in cases
of vaginismus, etc.

Superfœtation.—By superfœtation is meant the possibility of a woman, while pregnant, conceiving a second
time. In cases of superfœtation either two children are
born at the same time, one of which, however, is immature,
or two children are born at different times, both of which
are mature. Cases of superfœtation of the first kind
have been explained on the supposition that there has
been a twin conception, the development of one fœtus
having interfered in some way with that of the other.
That such cases of so-called superfœtation may be due
to repeated sexual intercourse and to successive con-
ceptions there can be no doubt, numerous cases having
occurred in which a negro woman, having had intercourse
successively with a black and a white man, gave birth in
due time to a black and a mulatto child. Indeed, it has
been stated upon good authority that in one instance
a Creole woman gave birth at one time to three children,
—white, brown, and black,—having all the features
of their respective parents.*

According to some authorities, double conception
occurs also in animals. Thus, if a bitch while in heat

* Beck: *op. cit.*, vol. I, pp. 317, 318; Dunglison: "Physiology,"
vol. II, p. 324.

receives two or three dogs of various species in succession, she may give birth to mongrel puppies, some partaking of the character of one dog, and others of the rest.*

Cases have also been reported in which the two sires have even been of different species—a mare, for example, covered successively by a horse and an ass, giving birth to a horse and a mule.† The possibility of the above occurring has been doubted by some biologists, though without apparently any good reason, since it only involves the condition that two ova were ready for impregnation at the moments that the mare was covered by the horse and the ass, the mare being fertile with both.

Cases of superfœtation of the second kind—that is, in which a woman gives birth to two mature children at an interval of three or four months—can, however, only be explained by supposing that the woman had sexual intercourse with one or two different men and conceived successively at about an equal interval of time of the two deliveries. As an example of such cases may be mentioned that of the wife of Raymond Villars, who gave birth on January 20, 1780, to a seven months' living child, which was nursed by another woman, the mother being unable at that time to furnish any milk. On July 6th of the same year the mother was delivered of a second living child, just five months and sixteen days after the birth of the first child. The milk now appeared and the mother was able to nourish her offspring. As the husband did not have intercourse with

* Ramsbotham: "Principles and Practice of Obstetric Medicine," etc., Phila., 1865, p. 463.

† Haller: "Elementa Physiologiæ," tomus VIII, p. 467; "Archiv Gén. de Médecine," tome XII, 1826, p. 125; tome XVII, 1828, p. 89; "Cyclop. of Anat. and Phys.," 1836–39, vol. II, p. 469.

his wife until twenty days after the first delivery, it is impossible to believe that the second child could have been conceived after the delivery of the first, as the first

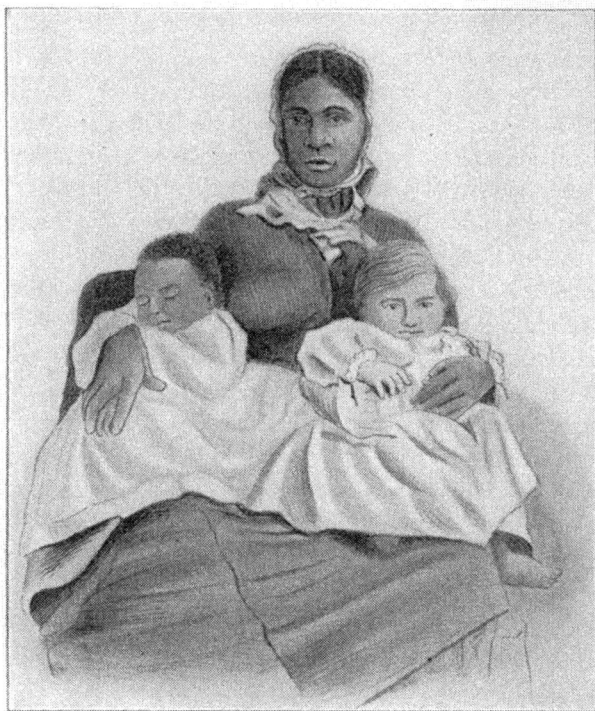

Fig. 31.—Mulatto mother with twins, one white and the other black (from a photograph after Flint). This case occurred on February 4, 1867, in New Kent County, Virginia, and was reported by Dr. J. H. Janeway, United States Surgeon.

child would then have been born four months and twenty days after conception and yet survive.

In another well-known case, a Mrs. T———, an Italian lady married to an Englishman, gave birth on November

12, 1807, to a healthy male child, which lived nine days, and on February 2, 1808, nearly three months after, to another male child, perfectly formed, which lived for three months, dying of measles.

Cases of superfœtation such as those just mentioned have been accounted for on the supposition that the uterus in the woman giving birth to two mature children at an interval of a few months was bifid, each uterus containing a fœtus more or less developed than the other. While a bifid uterus occurs occasionally in the human female,* as also normally in marsupial animals, like the kangaroo, it has been shown, when a woman so conditioned has become pregnant, that as a matter of fact only one uterus contained a fœtus.† One of the strongest objections that are urged against the possibility of superfœtation occurring in the normal female is that the presence of a fœtus of any size in the uterus would so block the passage of the spermatozoa as to render impossible the impregnation of a second ovum. It is obvious that if this objection has any weight, it will apply with equal force to the case of a bifid uterus with a single vagina, as well as to that of a single uterus. Further, even in those cases where the vagina has been found double, as well as the uterus, the reproductive apparatus being practically double, only one uterus contained a fœtus. Such cases throw no more light, therefore, upon the cause of superfœtation than do those of extra-uterine pregnancy. It must be admitted that such cases of superfœtation as the two

* Beck: *op. cit.*, vol. I, p 324.

† "Med.-Chir. Review," vol. xxiii, p. 234; "Guy's Hospital Reports," vol. vi, p. 551.

referred to above are rare, and that much difference of opinion still prevails among medical jurists as to whether there have ever occurred true cases of superfœtation, using that word in the sense in which it has been defined. Such being the case, the medical examiner should express himself with great caution *in foro,* as the majority of cases of alleged superfœtation originate, without doubt, either in fraud or in self-deception.

Paternity and Affiliation.—The question of paternity presents itself under various circumstances, as, for example, in cases of bastardy, where the alleged father is compelled to support the child, or where a bastard child claims to be the heir of an estate, or where a child is born ten months after a second marriage, the woman having married a second time within a month of the death of her first husband. In such cases the paternity is determined by the likeness of the child to the parent, the color, features, attitude, habits, gestures, voice, personal deformities being taken into consideration. Among such proofs of paternity, considerable importance, from time immemorial, has always been attached to the transmission of color. Thus, in the case of a white woman giving birth to a mulatto child, it would be undoubtedly inferred that the child's father was a black man—at least so thought the greatest of all poets:

> "Peace, tawny slave, half me and half thy dam.
> Did not thy nose bewray whose brat thou art,
> Had nature lent thee but thy mother's look,
> Villain, thou might'st have been an emperor!
> But where the bull and cow are both milk white,
> They never do beget a coal-black calf."

In certain cases questions of affiliation arise, as in the case of a woman having had intercourse with two men within a few days of each other and giving birth to a child, one of the men being affiliated as the father, rather than the other. In determining the paternity in such cases, the medical examiner should bear in mind that when a woman marries a second time, it is held by medical jurists that the children of such union may resemble the first husband rather than their own father. Though dead, yet speaking mysteriously from the grave, the peculiarities and even the diseases of the first husband may be transmitted to the children of his successor.* It should be mentioned, however, that the doctrine of telegony,†—of the offspring of the second husband inheriting the peculiarities, etc., of the first one,—though defended by Spencer, Romanes, has been much discredited in late years by biologists, among others, especially by Weismann.‡

Hermaphrodism.—Not infrequently, on account of divorce proceedings, questions in regard to legitimacy of offspring or capability of inheriting, voting, etc., the attention of the medical examiner is called to individuals in whom the sex is doubtful, or who are said to be hermaphrodites. While, as a general rule, there is no difficulty in distinguishing the sex in such cases, nevertheless, on account of the manner in which the external and internal generative organs develop in certain exceptional cases, it becomes very difficult, if not impossible, at least during life, to state positively whether an individual is a male or a female. At an early period of intra-uterine life—at six weeks or thereabouts—it is impossible to determine the sex of the embryo. The external organs

---

* Tidy: *op. cit.*, part ii, p. 73.

† τηλε, far off; γονος, offspring.

‡ Ewart, J. E.: "Penycuik Experiments," London, 1899. p. 165.

11

of generation are as yet undeveloped, and the internal organs consist (Fig. 32) of what may be called two indifferent bodies, the ducts of Müller and the Wolffian bodies. In case of such an embryo developing into a male, the two indifferent bodies will become testicles,

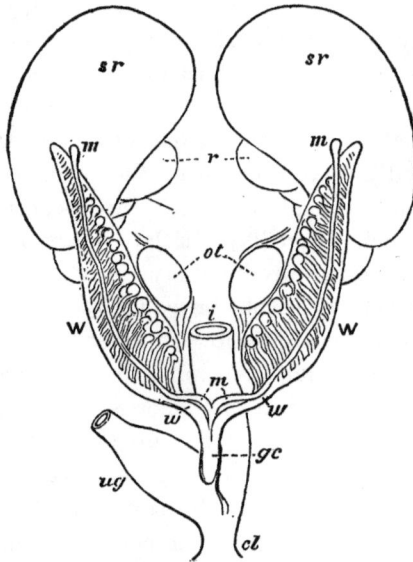

Fig. 32.—Diagram of the Wolffian bodies, Müllerian ducts, and adjacent parts previous to sexual distinction (as seen from before): *sr*, The suprarenal bodies; *r*, the kidneys; *ot*, common blastema of ovaries or testicles; *W*, Wolffian bodies; *w*, Wolffian ducts; *m m*, Müllerian ducts; *gc*, genital cord; *ug*, sinus urogenitalis; *i*, intestines; *cl*, cloaca (Quain).

which, in descending, push the abdominal walls ahead of them, giving rise in this way to the formation of the scrotum, which they ultimately occupy. The Wolffian bodies are transformed into the epididymis, vas deferens, etc., the ducts of Müller becoming atrophied.

On the other hand, should such an embryo develop into a female, the two indifferent bodies would become ovaries and remain in the abdominal cavity, and the ducts of Müller would be transformed into the vagina, uterus, and Fallopian tubes, the Wolffian bodies becoming atrophied. The penis and clitoris, developing later than the internal generative organs, consist essentially of the same parts, the only difference between them being due to the fact that the spongy body in the clitoris is undivided and does not inclose the urethra, as in the penis of the male, and that the two folds of skin which remain distinct, as the labia minora in the female, grow around and underneath, to form skin of the penis in the male.

That the clitoris and the penis are essentially homologous organs is still further proved by the fact that urination is accomplished by the clitoris in the female of lemurs, certain rodents, the hyæna crocuta, etc., exactly as by the penis in the male of the same species of animals and of man. Further, the two cutaneous folds constituting the labia majora of the female, in fusing together in the middle line, form the scrotum in the male.

Such being the development of the generative organs, it is readily seen, on the supposition that an individual is really a male, that, if the testicles in such a case were to remain in the abdominal cavity, the labia majora and minora failing at the same time to coalesce in the middle line, and the penis to remain undeveloped, such an individual might be easily mistaken for a female. On the other hand, if the clitoris, a highly erectile organ, was very much developed, as it is frequently, cases having been reported in which it was five inches long and one inch in diameter, and if it was used habitually for sexual intercourse, such an individual might be considered a male, it being supposed that the testicles had not descended; the absence of a scrotum being in that way explained.*

It is obvious, from what has been said, that a true human hermaphrodite—that is, a human creature in which a full, functionally complete set of organs are united in one individual—is a physical impossibility; for, even on the supposition that the Müllerian ducts and Wolffian bodies would be simultaneously transformed into vagina, uterus, epididymis, vasa deferentia, etc., one of the indifferent bodies into an ovary, the other into a testicle, which indeed has not infrequently occurred,† a penis would not be developed simultaneously with a clitoris, since, being essentially one and the same structure, one or the other is alone developed.

Whatever views may be held as to the possibility of true hermaphrodism occurring in the human species, as a matter of fact there is no authenticated case of any such creatures as a human hermaphrodite ever having existed; that is to say, of an individual who was capable of performing the sexual acts of either sex indifferently, and of impregnating the ova elaborated by the individual, by the spermatozoa produced by the same individual. Indeed, all the so-called hermaphrodites thus far examined have been shown sooner or later to be either androgynæ, manly women usually characterized by the presence of an elongated clitoris and other minor peculiarities, or androgyni, womanly men characterized by the absence, rudimentary condition, or malformation of the penis, with

* Beck: *op. cit.*, vol. I, pp. 169, 170, 172, 175.
† Tidy: *op. cit.*, part I, 330.

retention of the testicles in the inguinal canal or pelvic cavity.

It need hardly be added that, while there is no authenticated case of a true human hermaphrodite having ever existed, such a disposition of the generative apparatus not infrequently occurs among the lower animals, as in many of the mollusca, cestode and trematode worms, etc.

Doubtful Sex.—Not infrequently cases occur, as where an estate descends to the first-born male, in which the sex of the child born first is so doubtful that it can only be determined by a most thorough and expert examination, and in some cases not even then. In such cases the condition that confronts the medical examiner is not at all one of apparent hermaphrodism, of double sexual organs, but, on the contrary, the absence, more or less, of external or internal generative organs, or of both. Thus, for example, cases have been reported in which neither a penis nor a vagina was present;* where there was an absence of the lower part of the abdomen and of genital organs;† where a scrotum was present, but testicles and anus absent;‡ where there was a uterus, but no vagina,§ etc.

In cases where it is impossible for the medical examiner to say, at least during life, whether a child is male or female, there is nothing to do but to wait, since if the child survives till the age of puberty the secretion of healthy, active spermatozoa will establish the sex. In-

* "British Medical Journal," 1879, ii, p. 641.
† "Edinburgh Medical Journal," vol. xviii, p. 415
‡ "Edinburgh Medical Journal," vol xvi, p. 320.
§ "American Journal of the Medical Sciences," vol. lxiv, p. 575.

deed, the only reliable final test of sex is the power of producing spermatozoa or ova, the individual producing the former being a male, and the one producing the latter a female, irrespective of the presence, absence, or malformation of the external generative organs.

Monsters.—According to law, monsters are incapable of inheriting or transmitting property. A monster "hath no inheritable blood, and cannot be heir to any land, albeit it be brought forth in marriage."* It is very difficult, however, to say just what constitutes a monster, the law not defining the term. According to Blackstone, a monster is a creature "which hath not the shape of mankind"; but the great commentator leaves it conjectural as to what is meant by the expression "shape of mankind," and, further, what constitutes actual individuality, in the case of monsters. Whether the law will regard a creature with two heads, with or without two bodies, as two individuals, and every creature with one head, whether united to one or two bodies, a single one,† etc., it seems impossible to say. Indeed, the decisions of judges in cases involving the consideration of monsters have been so contradictory that it is questionable what the verdict would be in the case of a person who confessed, for example, to have drowned a child, regarding it as a monster, and ignorant apparently of having committed a crime. While such an act would be undoubtedly manslaughter, the absence of malice aforethought would probably lead to acquittal. Certainly, a legal

* Blackstone: "Commentaries on the Laws of England," London, 1829, book II, p. 246.

† St. Hilaire: "Histoire général et particulaire des Anomalies de l'Organisation chez l'Homme," Bruxelles, 1837, tome III, p. 331.

definition of a monster, and all that it implies, is still a great desideratum.

Cases involving the questions of **legitimacy** and **inheritance** are not often decided by the testimony of the medical expert alone, the evidence necessary to prove that a child is the offspring of adultery being of another character. In all such cases, however, questions may arise relating to the length of time in which gestation is shortened or prolonged, impotence, sterility, paternity, affiliation, superfœtation, doubtful sex, etc., the nature of which has just been considered. As regards the relation of premature birth to questions of legitimacy and inheritance, there is no doubt that eight, seven, and even six months' infants may survive.* It has been stated that in very exceptional instances even a fœtus but little over five months old may be viable. Indeed, it was so decided in the case of Cardinal Richelieu. There is no well-authenticated case, however, of a child of less than five months surviving twenty-four hours after its birth, and in only one instance did such a child live even that long.†

In cases, for example, where a living infant acquires the right of inheriting and transmitting property, the point that will have to be established is not whether the infant was viable in the sense that it would survive, but was it alive at the time of its birth, involving in turn the determination of what is meant by the expression being born alive.

---

* According to Haller: "Ante septimum mensem fœtus non potest superesse" ("Elementa Physiologiæ," tomus octavus, Lausanne, 1778, p. 423).

† Tidy: *op. cit.*, part II, p. 49.

Live Birth.—Considerable difference of opinion still exists, however, among medical jurists as to what constitutes a "live birth." The law demands, in order that a child be "born alive," that not only must the child be entirely expelled from the body of the mother, with the exception of the umbilical cord, but that the child must manifest at the moment of entire expulsion some sign or signs of life; must be, as it is defined, "viable," even though the child survive after birth but a moment, the term viable not being used medico-legally in the sense in which that word is ordinarily accepted—that is, capable of living.

Leaving out of consideration, however, what might be regarded as merely metaphysical distinctions, as a matter of fact that which constitutes a live birth will depend upon the significance attached to that expression by the law of the land, whatever that may be. In the United States and in England neither breathing nor crying is considered essential to establish the fact that a child was born alive. It is enough if the whole body has been brought into the world and the heart has throbbed, or if a movement of any kind has been made. In Scotland and Germany crying, and in France respiration, is requisite. That crying should not be regarded as indispensable in proving a live birth is obvious, since a child might be born alive and yet peradventure it might be born dumb.* The term *born alive* or *viable* being so understood, medico-legally, it might be stated with perfect propriety that a fœtus but six inches long, weighing only a few ounces, not more than four months old, and completely extruded from the mother, was born alive, was viable,—having

* Coke: "Institutes," Philadelphia, 1853, vol. i, 29*b*, 30*a*.

moved its arms and legs, opened its mouth, etc.,—though it died within half an hour of its birth. The law assumes that every child born in wedlock is legitimate unless it can be shown that the husband and wife had been separated for a longer time than that accepted as the average period of gestation, or that the husband was impotent. The difficulty, however, that would at once present itself in such a case is due to the impossibility of stating exactly what constitutes the accepted period of gestation. It is true that the average period of gestation is 280 days; nevertheless, there are authenticated cases, as already mentioned (page 151), in which gestation was prolonged to 325 days. Indeed, so great a difference of opinion still prevails among obstetricians as to what constitutes the normal duration of pregnancy, it continuing, according to high authorities,* even for twelve months, that the latter period has received the sanction of the Legislature of Pennsylvania as being legally the extreme limit of the duration of pregnancy. That is to say, if a married woman cannot prove that she has been in the company of her husband within twelve months next before the birth of the child, she is adjudged an adulteress and the child illegitimate, according to the fourth section of the Act of 1705.†

No period is fixed by English law beyond which a child, if born in wedlock, is deemed illegitimate, the question being left an entirely open one, and every case being decided upon its own merits.‡

* "British and Foreign Medical Review," vol. vi, p. 236; Meigs: "Obstetrics, the Science and Art," 1849, p. 194; Atlee: "American Journal of the Medical Sciences," October, 1846, p. 535.

† Wharton and Stillé: *op. cit.*, vol. iii, p. 49.

‡ Taylor: *op. cit.*, p. 640.

The Code Napoleon cuts the Gordian knot in regard to the normal period of pregnancy, in reference to cases of contested legitimacy, by fixing arbitrarily and unjustly the period of 180 days after marriage and 300 days after dissolution of marriage or non-access, between which periods children born may be regarded as legitimate. It must be admitted, however, that the strongest possible evidence would be required to prove the legitimacy of a child whose birth was shown not to have occurred until 325 days, and still more so a year, after the absence or death of the husband.

The law assumes that a child born in wedlock is legitimate unless it can be proved that the husband was impotent and sterile, by which it is meant that he was physically incapable, at the alleged period of conception, of begetting children, through inability of having sexual intercourse or of absence of spermatozoa from his semen.

It is important, with reference to the attaining of majority, that the exact day and hour of a child's birth be accurately noted—a person attaining a legal majority the first instant of the day before the twenty-first anniversary of his or her birthday, though forty-seven hours and fifty-nine minutes less than the complete number of days, counting by hours, on the principle that a part of a day is medico-legally equal to the whole of a day.* Further, as a child must be completely expelled from the body of its mother to constitute legally a live birth, it follows that the child begins to live at least legally at the moment of complete expulsion. Thus for example, the birthday of a child whose head left the mother at one minute to twelve on December 31, 1899, but whose

* Taylor: *op. cit.*, p. 599.

entire body did not follow until one minute past twelve on January 1, 1900, would be the latter date and not the former.*

Tenancy by Curtesy.—In cases where a husband acquires a life-interest in the estate of his wife, a child having been born during the life of the latter,—tenancy "by the curtesy of England,"† as it is called,—the medical examiner may be called upon to prove not only that the child was born alive, but also that it was born while its mother was living, that it was not a monster, etc., in order that the child may inherit.

With reference to the legal qualification of a child having been born during its mother's lifetime, the only difficulty that might present itself would be in the case of a child removed from its dead mother by the Cæsarean section, in which instance, if the letter of the law were carried out, the husband would be debarred from inheriting.

As the law regards a child as legitimate though not conceived in wedlock, the mother marrying afterward, and her condition being recognized by the husband at the time of the marriage, and as a child born after the death of its mother is legitimate, though the marriage-tie be dissolved by the death of the mother, it follows that a child, though conceived before marriage and born after the death of the mother,—that is, neither conceived nor born in wedlock,—would nevertheless be legally regarded as legitimate.

* Tidy: *op. cit.*, part ii, p. 294.
† Blackstone: *op. cit.*, vol. ii, p. 125.

CHAPTER XI.

Fœticide—Proofs of Development of Embryo—Formation of Placenta, of Moles—Of the Means of Producing Fœticide—Abortion from Natural Causes.

THE unlawful expulsion of the fœtus constitutes **fœticide,** or criminal abortion. By the term abortion or miscarriage is understood, medically, the expulsion of the fœtus before the sixth month of gestation—that is, before it would survive.* After this period the expulsion is called " premature labor." Legally, however, such a distinction is not made, the unlawful expulsion of the fœtus at any period of gestation being regarded as abortion. At one time the law also recognized a distinction between an abortion produced before and after quickening, the former crime being regarded as felony, the latter as murder, punishable by death,† it being arbitrarily assumed in English law that life does not begin until "an infant is able to stir in the mother's womb."‡

At the present time the criminality of the act is the same, whatever may be the period at which the abortion is committed. As it is perfectly evident that the fœtus must be alive at any period of intra-uterine development, the fœtus resulting from the development of a live ovum impregnated by a living spermatozoon, morally speaking,

* The fœtus, as we have already seen, only surviving in most exceptional cases if born before that period.

† Beck: *op. cit.,* vol. i, p. 462.

‡ Blackstone: *op. cit.,* vol. i, p. 129.

at least, the killing of a fœtus at any time before birth is as much murder as the killing of a child at any time after birth. Nevertheless, as a matter of fact, the crime of fœticide is regarded legally only as a felony, punishable by imprisonment; and although an extremely common crime, rarely becomes the subject of trial unless it involves the death of the mother, in which case it is murder or manslaughter, according to the law of the country or State in which the crime may have been committed.

Proofs of Fœticide.—The proofs that a criminal

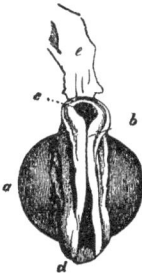

Fig. 33.—Human embryo, magnified ten times, about ten days old : *a*, Umbilical vesicle ; c, *b*, *d*, primitive spinal cord ; *e*, remains of amnion (Haeckel).

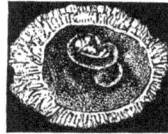

Fig. 34.—Human embryo, natural size, fourteen days old (Haeckel).

abortion has been committed are derived from the condition of the fœtus or fœtal remains, whether expelled from the uterus or still retained within it, and from the condition of the mother.

Development of the Human Embryo.—The human embryo,* at one of the earliest periods of development yet obtained,—that is, about from ten to fourteen days after conception,—consists (Fig. 33) of a tube, the primitive

* Haeckel: "Anthropogenie," vierte Auflage, erster Theil, Leipzig, 1891, S. 365.

neural canal, more or less open on top, from the under

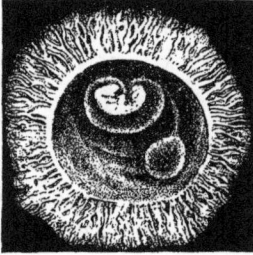

Fig. 35.—Human embryo, natural size, three weeks old (Haeckel).

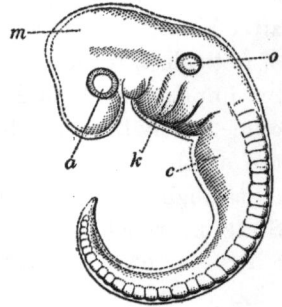

Fig. 36.—Human embryo, magnified, three weeks old: *a*, Eye; *m*, mid-brain; *o*, ear; *k*, visceral arches; *c*, heart (Haeckel).

part of which hangs a globular-like bag. The latter, through subsequent constriction, divides into an upper

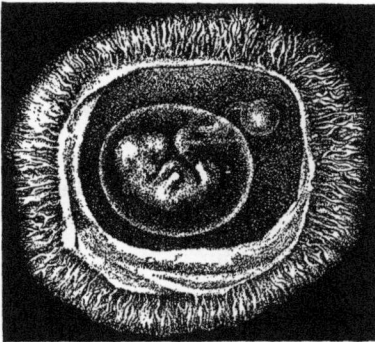

Fig. 37.—Human embryo, natural size, six weeks old (Haeckel).

and lower portion continuous with each other, which become respectively the primitive alimentary canal and the umbilical vesicle.

The embryo, not longer than one-twelfth of an inch, and inclosed within the amniotic folds, does not lie naked within the uterus, but within the zona pellucida (Fig. 34) or the original membrane which inclosed the yelk, or the contents of the egg. The zona pellucida, being covered, however, with little villus-like processes, is known now and henceforth as the chorion. By the twenty-first day of uterine life the embryo (Figs. 35, 36), having attained a length of about one-sixth of an inch, rudimentary eyes and ears, the mouth, three cerebral vesicles, bronchial arches and clefts, umbilical vesicle, allantois, and amnion are all developed. At the end of the first month, the embryo, being one-half of an inch long and weighing perhaps about twenty grains, is still further developed and is provided with rudimentary limbs. By the end of the sixth week the embryo (Fig. 37) has grown larger, and the limbs are better developed, attaining at the end of the second month (Fig. 38) a length of one inch, and weighing about one-eighth of an ounce. The fingers and toes are also now indicated, and ossification has begun in the lower

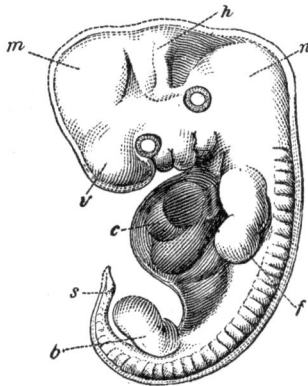

Fig. 38.—Human embryo, magnified, eight weeks old : v, Fore-brain; m, mid-brain ; h, hind-brain ; n, after-brain ; c, heart; f, upper extremity ; b, lower extremity ; s, tail (Haeckel).

jaw, clavicle, ribs, and vertebral bodies. At the third month the embryo (Fig. 39) is about two to two and a half inches long, and weighs about one ounce; the sex can usually be distinguished by the external genitalia, and the placenta is beginning to be formed.

Formation of the Placenta.—It will be observed that the villous processes of the chorion, which have hitherto covered the latter membrane throughout its whole extent.

are now limited to that portion of it in contact with the *decidua serotina* or that part of the hypertrophied mucous membrane of the uterus into which the villous processes of the chorion still remaining insinuate themselves. The fusion of the two constitutes the *placenta* (Plate 3, Fig. 1).

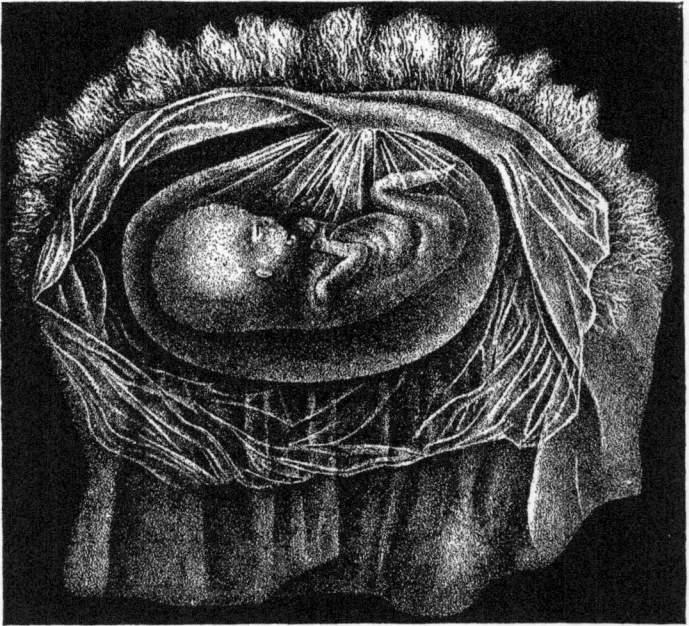

Fig. 39.—Human embryo, natural size, three months old (Haeckel).

Of the remaining portion of the hypertrophied mucous membrane of the uterus, that part which ultimately grows around the ovum is known as the *decidua reflexa*, and that in contact with the wall of the uterus, the *decidua vera*.

PLATE 3.

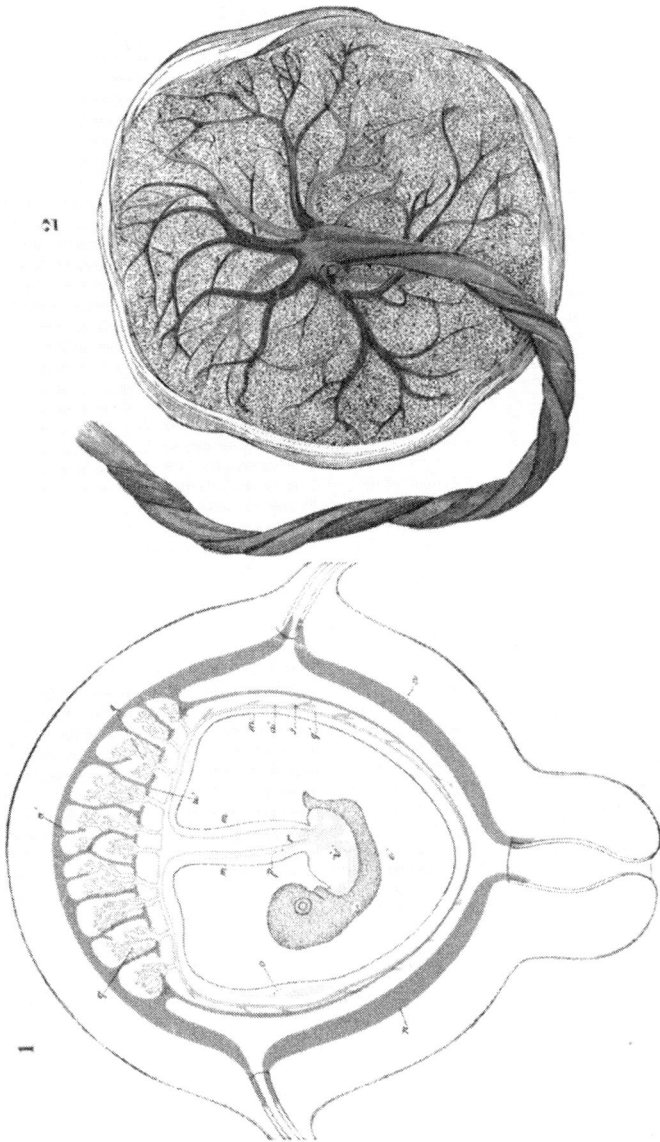

1. Diagrammatic Section of Uterus, Embryo, and Placenta: a, a', allantois transformed into chorion; c', embryo; i, rudimentary intestine; m m, amnion; n, decidua vera; n', decidua serotina; o, umbilical vesicle; p, pedicle of umbilical vesicle; q, villi of the chorion forming foetal portion of placenta; q', villi of the chorion imbedded in decidua reflexa and in the process of disappearing; r, pedicle of allantois; r', lacunæ of decidua serotina forming maternal portion of placenta (Longet)   2. Portion of the Umbilical Cord and the Fœtal Surface of the Human Placenta in the Normal State.

The villous processes of the chorion, when examined with the microscope, present so characteristic an appearance (Fig. 40) that their presence may be accepted as positive proof of the existence of the embryo, even if not a trace of the latter be found.* The general appearance of the villous process is like that of a sea-weed, originating in the chorion by a trunk which divides and subdivides into filamentous branches, swollen here and there, terminating in rounded bulbous extremities, and consisting internally of a finely granular substance containing nuclei. At first the villous processes of the chorion are without blood-vessels, but with the development of the allantois they become vascular through prolongation of the terminal allantoic vessels, which are disposed in loops. The placenta (Plate 3, Fig. 2), or afterbirth, consisting essentially of the interlacement of the blood-vessels of the embryo with those of the mother, is a flattened, fleshy, vascular, dish-like mass, round or ovoid in shape and with a diameter of from six to eight inches. It is the organ by means of which food and oxygen are conveyed from the blood

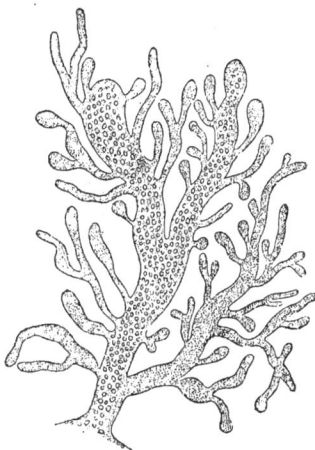

Fig. 40. — Villous processes of human chorion, ramified extremity ; from a three months' fœtus, magnified thirty diameters (Dalton).

* Dalton, John C.: "Human Physiology," seventh edition, Philadelphia, 1882, p. 647.

12

of the mother to that of the embryo. The process by which this is accomplished is, however, by osmosis, as there is never at any period of gestation an anastomosis of the maternal and fœtal blood-vessels.

Such being the structure and development of the placenta, it is evident that, just in proportion as the fœtal and maternal portions of the placenta become more and more intimately fused together, the greater will be the difficulty experienced and risk run in the expulsion of the fœtus from the uterus. It is for this reason that an abortion committed after the third month of gestation may be attended with such fatal consequences, the hemorrhage resulting from the rupture of the blood-vessels being at times very great. Indeed, at a late period of gestation the maternal blood-vessels become dilated into great sinuses, veritable blood lakes. On the other hand, if gestation has not advanced beyond the third month, the embryo may, under certain circumstances, be expelled entire from the uterus, very much as a glove is removed from the fingers, without any serious consequences.

Subsequent Changes Undergone by the Human Embryo.—The subsequent changes undergone by the embryo during the last six months of pregnancy are of interest, medico-legally, as enabling the examiner to state the probable age of a fœtus obtained from a supposed case of abortion. At the fourth month the fœtus is five to six inches long and weighs about three ounces, the umbilical cord measuring about seven inches in length. At the fifth month the fœtus has attained a length of six to seven inches, weighs from five to seven ounces, and is covered with the vernix caseosa; the hair of the head and body, or lanugo, is quite distinct, and the umbilical cord is about twelve inches long. If abortion occurs at this period of gestation, the membranes are first ruptured, and then the fœtus is expelled from the uterus. At the sixth month of pregnancy the fœtus varies in length from nine to ten inches, weighs a pound or more, and meconium is usually found in the intestines.

At the end of the seventh month the fœtus is usually fourteen inches long, weighs two and a half to three pounds, the eyes are open, the membrane of the pupil is disappearing, one testicle has descended into the inguinal canal. If the child should be born at this period, the arms and legs will be bent in the position they assumed in the womb, and it will be viable. At the eighth month the fœtus is sixteen inches long, weighs between three and four pounds; the skin has become thicker, and is covered with fine soft hair; one testicle, usually the left, has descended into the scrotum. At the end of the ninth month, or at full term, the fœtus varies in length from eighteen to twenty-one inches, weighing on an average seven pounds, the umbilical cord or funis being about the same length as the child's body. Some rare cases, however, have been reported in which the cord measured at full term not only fifty-nine and a half inches, but even sixty-nine inches.* The intestines are nearly filled with meconium; the bladder contains urine; both testicles have descended into the scrotum.

As aiding in determining the age of the fœtus, it may be mentioned that at full term the umbilical cord is usually inserted about eight to ten lines below the center of the body; whereas, at an earlier period of gestation, the

* Wharton and Stillé: *op. cit.*, vol. iii, p. 118.

point of insertion is at the middle of the body. The general development of the brain, the extent to which the cerebellum is covered by the cerebrum, the particular fissures that are present, will also serve to determine the age of the fœtus. The importance of the presence or absence of an osseous deposit in the inferior epiphysis of the femur has already been referred to (page 55).

It should be mentioned, in connection with the subject of the length and weight of the fœtus at full term, that these may vary considerably.* Thus, for example, it is well known that children have been born at full term who measured as much as twenty-four and even thirty-two inches, and who weighed as much as seventeen and three-quarters pounds † and eighteen pounds and two ounces,‡ respectively. On the other hand, children at full term not infrequently weigh only from four to six pounds. There is usually no difficulty experienced in recognizing an embryo *in situ*, or even amid the contents expelled from a uterus in cases of abortion, unless the latter be committed in the very early periods of gestation.

Moles.—Under certain circumstances the medical examiner may be called upon to determine whether peculiar growths, either formed in the uterus or expelled from it, are polypi or membranous in character, as due to dysmenorrhœa, or what are known as *moles*.§ It is most

* As to variability in size and weight presented by the fœtus at different periods of intra-uterine life, compare Casper, vol. iii, pp. 15–17; Guy and Ferrier, p. 88; Tidy, part ii, p. 59; Wharton and Stillé, vol. iii, p. 75; Woodman and Tidy, pp. 647, 712.

† Owens: "Lancet," December, 1838, p. 477.

‡ Meadows: "Medical Times and Gazette," August 4, 1860, p. 105.

§ Montgomery: *op. cit.*, pp. 255, 269, 326, 353.

important that the true nature of the latter, when present, should be recognized, as moles, being due to disease of the placenta or of the fœtal membranes, are as much proof of a pregnancy having existed as the presence of the embryo itself. Moles, when due to disease of the placenta, are either fleshy or fatty. A fleshy mole consists of layers of a fibrinous material inclosing a cavity in which the remains of the fœtus are sometimes formed. While the cause of fleshy moles is obscure in some instances, they appear usually to be due to hemorrhage into the chorion. A fatty mole differs more particularly from a fleshy one in that a fatty degeneration is an accompaniment of the early death of the fœtus. The hydatidiform or vesicular mole is due to the villous processes of the chorion becoming infiltrated with serum, and hanging in masses like bunches of grapes. A true hydatid—that is, a helminth of the uterus—is exceedingly rare. Indeed, only two cases of such have been reported as occurring in the human female.*

The **proofs of an abortion** having been committed, as derived from an examination of the mother, are not very positive, if the act has been performed at an early period of pregnancy. The hemorrhage and relaxed condition of the vagina, for example, and the somewhat dilated condition of the os uteri, might be attributed to menstruation. If the pregnancy was, however, far advanced at the time of the occurrence of the abortion, the proofs will usually be sufficiently strong to establish the fact. It is far more difficult, therefore, for a woman to conceal her pregnancy and the fact that an abortion had been committed to save her from exposure, at a late period of gestation than at an early one. If death follows within three days after abor-

* Tidy: *op. cit.*, part II, p. 121.

tion, the post-mortem examination will generally establish the fact that an abortion was committed. If several weeks, however, have elapsed, little or nothing will be learned by the autopsy, as the parts involved will have usually re-assumed by that time their usual condition.

In every case of fœticide the vagina and uterus should be examined most carefully for metritis and marks of violence which might have been produced by the use of instruments. Wounds of the vagina would rather indicate that they had not been made by a professional abortionist, but by one who was inexperienced in such work and who had been rendered nervous in attempting to perform the operation. If the neck of the uterus or its fundus be found perforated, or the placenta wounded, the inference to be drawn would be that pointed instruments had been used, though not necessarily, since fatal wounds have been also inflicted by blunt instruments. The most common causes of death in cases of abortion as produced by instrumental violence are hemorrhage and peritonitis. The stomach and intestines should also be carefully examined in cases of fœticide, as they present, not infrequently, evidence that irritant poisons have been taken. Remains of cantharides, tops of savin, ergot, may be found; or the oils of savin, tansy pennyroyal, may be recognized by their odor or by appropriate chemical means, such as distillation, etc. The shape and size of the uterus should be carefully noted in cases of fœticide, as they enable the examiner to determine approximately at least the age of the fœtus.

Changes in Size of Uterus.—The normal uterus in the unimpregnated condition measures about two and a half inches in length, one inch and three-quarters in breadth, and one inch thick. As pregnancy advances, the uterus increases gradually in size—very little change being noticeable, however, during the first month. During the second month the increase is considerable. By the end of the third month it has attained a length of five inches, including one inch for the cervix. At the end of the fourth month the uterus is five inches long from the fundus to the beginning of the cervix, and at the end of the fifth, sixth, and seventh month it is six, seven, and eight inches long, respectively. At eight months the uterus varies in length from nine to nine and a half inches, and at nine months from between ten and a half to twelve inches in its total length. While the thickness of the walls of the uterus at full term is about the same as that in the unimpregnated condition, or from one-third to two-thirds of an inch, within a few hours after delivery they may become, through contraction, at least two inches thick.

The **changes in the shape of the uterus** presented at different periods of gestation are also very characteristic. From being flat and pyriform, the uterus, after impregnation, becomes globular; the cervix, also, as already mentioned (page 147), gradually shortens, according to most obstetricians, until at full term it has disappeared entirely, the form of the uterus being then ovoid. After delivery at full term the uterus begins usually to contract, its size being reduced within two days to six inches in length and four in breadth. By the end of the first week it has so contracted as to measure usually from five to six inches in length. At the end of the second week the uterus is about four inches long and one and a half inches broad. By the end of the second month it has returned to its normal size.

In those cases, however, in which death occurring at full term is due to hemorrhage, no contraction of the uterus will have taken place. If the woman, however, has survived for a few days, the uterus will be found more or less contracted. During pregnancy the round ligaments and Fallopian tubes increase in size and become more vascular; the broad ligaments are gradually effaced through the great development.

Means of Producing Fœticide.—Among the means first tried by women to bring on a miscarriage may be mentioned the effects of violence, such as submitting to a severe beating, jumping from high places, as tops of fences, gates, etc., venesection, emetics, and drastic cathartics.* As a general rule, however, except in the case of very feeble or weakly women, or in those who are predisposed to miscarriage, such measures fail to produce an abortion. The emmenagogues, or the drugs known popularly as abortives, are then next resorted to, on account of the power they are supposed to possess of inducing uterine contractions and of thus causing the expulsion of the fœtus. Among these, the ones most commonly used are ergot or spurred rye, cotton-root, savin, or the tops of the Juniperus sabina, tansy, pennyroyal, and rue. But large doses may be taken of these drugs without causing uterine contraction, while the oils of savin and tansy have frequently caused death, through gastritis or peritonitis being produced by their irritant properties.

All such means having failed to produce an abortion, instrumental violence, as a last resource, is made use of as the only certain means of inducing uterine contractions

* Tardieu: "Etude Médico-legale sur l'Avortement," troisième edition, Paris, 1688, pp. 28, 99.

and of so insuring the expulsion of the fœtus. The rupture of the fœtal membranes, however skilfully performed, is a most dangerous operation, always liable to be followed by the most serious, if not fatal, consequences, death being frequently caused, as already mentioned, by either hemor-rhage or peritonitis. When the operation is performed by a professional abortionist, long, narrow, sharp-pointed in-struments are made use of; but when self-inflicted, which is not infrequently the case, the woman uses any articles that may serve her purpose, such as knitting-needles, pen-holders, long wires, glove-stretchers, whalebones, branches of trees, pieces of wood, syringes, etc.*

Abortion from Natural Causes.—It should be men-tioned, in connection with the subject of fœticide, that abor-tion very frequently results from natural causes. Indeed, with some women it appears to be habitual, abortion occurring at every pregnancy, especially in the early months of gestation, though every effort has been made to prevent it. As might be expected, the tendency to abortion is most marked at the menstrual periods. Predisposition to abortion appears to be due to causes which affect the mother, such as syphilis, smallpox, albuminuria, etc., or those which affect the child, as death of the ovum, disease of the placenta. Advantage is no doubt often taken of this natural tendency to abort by producing abortion criminally. As natural abortion usually occurs at about the third or fourth month of pregnancy, and as this period is also the one at which a criminal operation is performed, the fact that the fœtus comes away entire would indicate that abortion was due to natural causes, or at least not to

* Wharton and Stillé: *op. cit.*, vol. iii, pp. 66–70; Beck: *op. cit.*, vol. i, p. 486.

instrumental violence. If, however, the fœtus be expelled first and the ruptured membranes afterward, the conclusion would be that instruments had been used.

Abortion may sometimes be feigned by women, in order to extort money on the charge of seduction and consequent pregnancy. The examination of the woman will usually be sufficient, under such circumstances, to disprove the charge. The criminality of fœticide is not excused by the fact that the woman was not pregnant, or by the fact that the pregnancy was extra-uterine. Under certain circumstances it may become necessary to perform an abortion, as in cases, for example, where the deformity of the pelvis makes the delivery of a living child at full term a physical impossibility. In all such cases the attending physician should insist upon a consultation being held; and the patient and her family should be fully informed as to the nature of the case before so serious an operation is undertaken.

CHAPTER XII.

Infanticide—Importance of Corpus Delicti; History of Infanticide —Appearance of Infant Born Alive at Full Term—Means of Determining whether Child Has Breathed—Docimasia Pulmonum— Objections to Hydrostatic Test—Docimasia Circulationis—Size of Liver and Contents of Stomach in New-born Child—Examination of Mother—Signs of Recent Delivery—Means by which Infanticide is Committed.

By infanticide is meant, medico-legally, the murder of the new-born child, it being immaterial whether the child is murdered immediately or a few days after its birth. To be born alive implies, medico-legally, as already mentioned (page 168), complete expulsion of a living child from the mother; a child, for example, not born alive if any portion of it, except the umbilical cord, is retained within the vulva. By this absurd interpretation of law, utterly inconsistent with well-established physiological facts and even with common sense, the destruction of a living child, if only partly born, does not constitute murder. Thus, in a well-known trial that occurred in England (Dorset Lent Assizes, 1845), the defendant was acquitted of the charge of murder notwithstanding that it was in evidence that he had killed an infant whilst it was being born by cutting its head off, the learned judge drawing a fine distinction between physiological and medical life. "Medically," said he, "this might be a live child; but legally it was not one, for in law the birth of the child must be complete." * Other such

* Tidy: *op. cit.*, part II, p. 249.

cases might be mentioned in which the defendant has been acquitted of the charge of infanticide, though guilty, upon exactly the same grounds.

Establishment of Corpus Delicti.—There are no classes of cases which demand the consideration of the medical jurist that illustrate more forcibly the importance of establishing the corpus delicti than those of infanticide. Indeed, many cases have occurred in which, through the neglect of the identification of the deceased infant, the prosecution has failed, on trial, to convict the person accused of having committed the crime. Of many such instances that might be mentioned, the following, to which the attention of the author was recently called, will suffice as as illustration: Two infants were found by a policeman in an alley, one of which had been undoubtedly murdered; the other had died a natural death. Neither of them was, however, properly identified by those to whom had been assigned the duty of officially investigating the cause of death. The result of such neglect, as might have been anticipated by those familiar with the methods of criminal prosecution, was that at the very beginning of the trial the prosecution failed to show that the infant for whose death the supposed mother was held was the identical infant that had been murdered, and not the infant that had died a natural death. In other words, for aught that the prosecution could prove, it was just as likely, through the want of the establishment of the corpus delicti, that the infant that had died a natural death was the child of the defendant as the infant that had been murdered. The case, of course, fell through, and the defendant was acquitted, though possibly guilty.

The law assumes, until it is proved to the contrary, that every child is born dead, on account of the fact that so many children are brought into the world who are either dead or die shortly after birth. Inasmuch as this is the law, the prosecution, and not the defendant, must prove that the infant alleged to have been murdered was born alive. For this reason great difficulty is usually experienced in convicting a woman charged with the crime of infanticide. Apart from this difficulty, she is often delivered in the absence of witnesses, or the child is concealed or destroyed. The jury also often sympathizes to such an extent with a woman accused of this crime that conviction cannot easily be secured. Infanticide is, therefore, at the present day a common crime, though much less so than in former times.

It is well known that among the Jews even as late as the Babylonian captivity infanticide was very common * notwithstanding that the crime had been denounced by their God.† In Persia it was a common occurrence to bury children alive in order to get rid of them.‡ In ancient Greece, with perhaps the exception of Thebes, infanticide was not only permitted, but actually enforced by law. In Sparta, for example, every weak or deformed child was thrown into a deep cavern at the foot of Mount Tayetus, it being held that its life would be of no advantage to any one.§

Such a revolting practice as infanticide was defended, strange as it may appear, by the most distinguished among the Greeks, as by Aristotle in his treatise upon government and Plato in his "Republic," and referred to as an everyday occurrence by the poets Euripides in "Ion," Sophocles in the "Œdipus Tyrannus," etc. At no time, however,

* Jeremiah, 19: 5; 32: 35; Ezekiel, 16: 20, 21; 22: 37, 39.
† Leviticus, 20: 1.   ‡ Herodotus, "Polymnia," 114.
§ Plutarch's "Lives," translated by Langhorne, vol. i, p. 142.

was the practice of infanticide so common as when Rome
had reached the pinnacle of its grandeur, the Roman empire, according to its great historian, being stained with
the blood of infants,* notwithstanding that ecclesiastical
writers like Justin Martyr and Tertullian, and even the
Latin poets themselves, had exposed and denounced the
crime—among the latter the greatest satirist of his day,
and indeed of all time.

> "Yet these, though poor, the pain of child-bed bear,
> And without nurses their own infants rear.
> You seldom hear of the rich mantle spread
> For the babe born in the great lady's bed,
> Such is the power of herbs; such arts they use,
> To make them barren, or their fruit to lose." †

A Roman father had but to leave his child on the ground
where the midwife, according to custom, had just placed
it at birth if he did not wish to rear it; on the other hand
picking it up by the act of "tollere liberum" and handing
it to the mother or nurse if he wished it to live.   And yet,
among contemporary Goths and Germans, to their credit
be it said, though the Romans stigmatized them as bar-
barians, infanticide, though prevalent, was not sanctioned
among them, at least by law.   Indeed, it was not until the
accession of Constantine that any systematic effort was
made to suppress infanticide by law, and which was only
finally accomplished during the reigns of his successors,
Valentinian, Valens, and Gratian.   Infanticide is still a
very common crime in China, India, and in the South Sea

* Gibbon: "The History of the Decline and Fall of the Roman
Empire," vol. viii, p. 51.

† Juvenal: Sat. vi, 591, Dryden's translation.

Islands, the number of infants murdered being almost incredible.*

The law assuming, as just mentioned, that all children are born dead, it becomes a matter of practical importance for the medical examiner to be able to distinguish a child born alive from the stillborn.

Appearance of an Infant Born Alive at Full Term.— In infanticide the child is generally born at full term, the general appearance presented being as follows: Remains of the vernix caseosa or sebaceous matter are usually found behind the ears and under the armpits; the hair is dry and clean; the eyes are half open, and cannot be kept closed; the ears do not lie close to the head; the caput succedaneum, or swelling on the back of the head, is well marked; the thorax is distinctly arched, and the diaphragm much depressed. A dead-born child is usually covered with the vernix caseosa; the hair is agglutinated; the eyes are closed; the ears lie close to the head; the thorax is flattened and unexpanded; the lungs lie in the posterior part of the thorax, are granular, and do not crepitate upon pressure.†

In case of the death of the fœtus some time before birth, the body will be found flaccid and flattened, as if it had been macerated; the cuticle may be more or less detached, especially upon the abdomen; the head lies flat, howsoever it may be placed, the cranial bones moving readily upon one another, the cellular tissue infiltrated with bloody serum.

The proofs of a child having breathed, and therefore of

---

* For a more detailed account of the history of infanticide the reader is referred to an admirable article in Beck, *op. cit.*, vol. I, p. 427.

† Wharton and Stillé: *op. cit.*, vol. III, p. 80.

having lived, in a physiological sense at least, though not necessarily of having been born alive in a legal one,—that is, after complete expulsion from the body of the mother,— are derived from the condition of the respiratory, circulatory, and abdominal organs.

Means of Determining whether the Child Has Breathed.—While the vaulted character of the thorax, the comparative depression of the diaphragm, the relation of the larynx to the epiglottis, the situation, volume, color, consistence, absolute or relative weight, the specific gravity of the lungs, may all be important under certain circumstances in enabling the examiner to determine whether an infant has breathed, nevertheless the hydrostatic test is the only one that can be relied upon, and even that with certain qualifications, to be presently mentioned.

Docimasia Pulmonum Hydrostatica.—The principle of the hydrostatic test is based upon the fact that while the lungs of an infant that have been aerated will float when placed in water on account of the inspired air, those of an infant that have not been aerated will sink. · To apply the hydrostatic test, the lungs should be removed from the chest of an infant and put in a sufficiently capacious vessel containing distilled water at 60° F. If the lungs float upon the surface of the water, that will prove that they have been aerated. It is desirable also that each lung should be divided into a dozen or more pieces, compressed, and then tested separately in the same manner. If after compression all the pieces float, very complete aeration would be indicated. It must be admitted that the hydrostatic test, while it serves to determine whether the lungs of the infant had or had not been aerated, does not necessarily prove that the child had breathed, still less had been alive in a medico-legal sense, although it may establish a strong presumption of the fact; for it is well known that in certain rare cases of tedious labors, or when the obstetrician had occasion to perform version, after the rupture of the membranes and the dilatation of the mouth of the uterus, the head of the infant was, nevertheless, retained sufficiently long in the uterus or vagina for the infant not only to breathe, but even to cry loud enough (vagitus uterinus and vaginalis) to be heard by several persons in the room,* though subsequently born dead. It is not impossible, also, though improbable, that the air found in the lungs of the infant may have been artificially introduced, developed through putrefaction, or be emphysematous in nature. Apart from the difficulty, if not impossibility, of artificially inflating the lungs of an infant *in situ*, in cases of infanticide there would be no motive for any one to attempt to do so, unless it were the obstetrician or the mother, the object being to save life; or very improbably by some one to maliciously criminate another. Certainly, nothing of the kind would be attempted by the defendant in case of infanticide, since the absence of air from the lungs would favor the idea that the child had been born dead and not alive.

Further, lungs inflated artificially differ very much in their color from those inflated naturally, the latter being of a pale red, passing insensibly into blue, or presenting the characteristic marble appearance of irregular, light red spots upon a blue-red ground.

As a general rule, there is no great difficulty experienced in determining whether the buoyancy of a lung is due to air inspired or to gases developed within it through

* Wharton and Stillé; *op. cit.*, vol. III, p. 90,

13

putrefaction, since the air in the latter case is not found in the air-vesicles of the lungs, but in the cellular tissue and in the form of large bubbles, which disappear completely under pressure. Moreover, lungs in a state of putrefaction differ in appearance very much from healthy lungs, being greenish-yellow in color, having but little consistence, and emitting a fetid odor. It may be mentioned, also, in this connection, that as the lungs of the infant do not putrefy so rapidly as the other organs, if these organs are found undecomposed, then any buoyancy exhibited by the lungs could not be due to putrefaction. As there is not one well-authenticated case of emphysema ever having spontaneously developed in the lungs of an infant, the objection that the air in the lungs could be developed in this way is without foundation.* On the other hand, it may be objected that the fact that the lungs sink when immersed in water does not necessarily prove that the infant had not breathed, since the unaerated condition of the lungs might be due to disease. While it is true that the density of the lungs will be so much increased by pneumonia or congestion that they will sink in water, these diseases, as well as pulmonary apoplexy, tumors, fluid in the pleuræ, occur so rarely in newborn children that but little importance need be attached to such an objection.

It need hardly be added that the condition of atelectasis pulmonum, or imperfect expansion of the lungs in the fœtus, is not one of disease, but normally incidental to immature development.

Notwithstanding that the value of the hydrostatic test has been questioned, that it cannot be expected

* Casper: *op. cit.*, vol. iii, p. 72.

to prove absolutely that the child has breathed, still less been born alive, medico-legally, yet if the lungs of an infant do float in water, the medical examiner will be warranted, under ordinary circumstances, in stating that the infant had breathed, and in all probability had been born alive.

Docimasia Circulationis.—The test of an infant having been born alive, or rather of having breathed, based upon the changes undergone by the heart and certain blood-vessels, after respiration has been established, is of rather limited application, as will become apparent when the differences between the fœtal and adult circulations are considered.

Fœtal Circulation.—The principal peculiarities in which the circulation of the fœtus differs from that of the adult are that little or no blood flows through the lungs of the fœtus, the placenta being the organ by means of which the blood is aerated, and that the right side of the heart communicates with the left, the blood being, therefore, neither arterial nor venous, as in the adult, but mixed. In the fœtus (Plate 4) part of the blood flows directly from the right auricle through the foramen ovale into the left auricle, instead of indirectly by the right ventricle, pulmonary artery, lungs, and pulmonary veins; part of the blood from the right ventricle through the pulmonary artery by the ductus arteriosus into the aorta. Further, the blood flows in the fœtus from the placenta by the umbilical vein, and its continuation, the ductus venosus, to the vena cava and to the right side of the heart, and thence through the latter as just described, little or none going to the lungs, to the aorta, and so back by the umbilical arteries to the placenta.

Such being the main features of the fœtal circulation, with the inspiration of air and the separation of the infant from the placenta by division of the umbilical cord the foramen ovale closes, the umbilical vessels, the ductus arteriosus, and the ductus venosus shrivel up, and, ceasing to be pervious, become fibrous cords. The blood then flows through the heart and lungs, and the adult circulation is established.

Under ordinary circumstances, if the foramen ovale, ductus venosus, and ductus arteriosus are found open, the examiner would be warranted in stating that the fœtus had not been born alive, and that, therefore, in all probability, if any crime had been committed, it would be that of fœticide, and not of infanticide. Not infrequently, however, several days or even weeks may elapse before the blood ceases to flow through these vessels, and the foramen ovale may remain, under certain circumstances, open through life. On the other hand, the ductus venosus has been found closed in an infant born dead, and both the ductus arteriosus and the foramen ovale closed in one that lived only a quarter of an hour. It is obvious, therefore, that too much importance must not be attached to the open or closed condition of the heart and vessels as evidence of the infant having been born dead or alive. The drying up of the part of the umbilical cord remaining attached to the umbilicus after division, that usually takes place within two or three days after delivery, together with its subsequent separation and cicatrization, may be regarded as proof of the child having been born alive, since, although the cord withers and dries up in a child born dead as well as in one born alive, it always remains attached in the former to the umbilicus, never separating spontaneously.

PLATE 4.

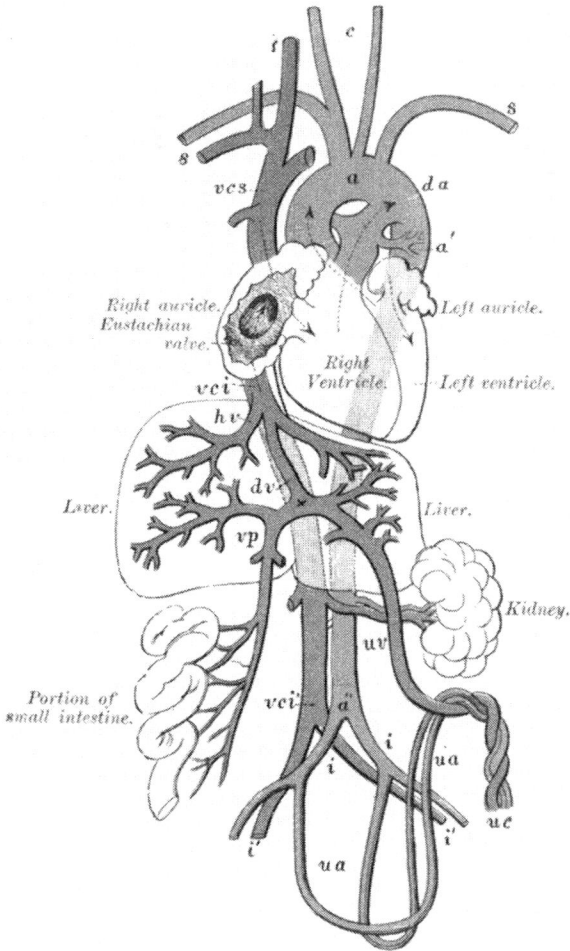

Diagrammatic View of Fœtal Circulation: *a*, arch of the aorta; *a'*, its dorsal part; *a''*, lower end; *vcs*, superior vena cava; *vci*, inferior vena where it joins the right auricle; *vci'*, its lower end; *s*, subclavian vessels; *j*, right jugular vein; *c*, common carotid arteries; four curved dotted arrow-lines are carried through the aortic and pulmonary opening, and the auriculo-ventricular orifices; *da*, opposite to the one passing through the pulmonary artery, marks the place of the ductus arteriosus; a similar arrow-line is shown passing from the vena cava inferior through the fossa ovalis of the right auricle, and the foramen ovale into the left auricle; *hv*, the hepatic veins; *vp*, vena portæ; × to *vci*, the ductus venosus; *uv*, the umbilical vein; *ua*, umbilical arteries; *uc*, umbilical cord cut short; *i, i'*, iliac vessels.

Liver and Contents of the Stomach in a New-born Child.—The liver of the foetus is larger than that of a recently born infant, and that of the infant is larger than that of an eight or ten months old child. Too much importance, however, must not be attached to the size of the liver as positive proof of the infant having lived after birth, since the difference in the size of the liver in a recently born child, as compared with its size at earlier or later stages of development, is only relative. The presence of milk or of farinaceous and saccharine articles of food in the stomach or intestine of an infant would be strong evidence that it had lived some time after birth. Unfortunately, the remains of food are not very frequently found in the alimentary canal of infants alleged to have been destroyed. In certain cases of infanticide it may become of importance to determine the age of the new-born child and the time that has elapsed since its death. Its age can approximately be determined by ascertaining whether it presents all the characters of a fully matured foetus that have already been described. It is not often possible to state exactly the time elapsing between the birth and the death of an infant, as so many conditions have to be taken into consideration, such as the season of the year, the temperature, the character of the place, and the surroundings of the infant.

Examination of the Mother; Signs of Recent Delivery.—In all cases of infanticide the reputed mother should be examined as well as the infant. The examination should be made as soon as possible, for, if delayed beyond a week or ten days, the woman may have so recovered as to present no signs of having been recently delivered. Should the examination be made within three or four days after delivery, pallor of the face and weakness will be noticed; the skin will be found moist, soft, and relaxed; the eyes somewhat sunken. The pulse is soft and usually quick. The uterus can be felt through the wall of the abdomen, which feels soft, and presents transverse livid lines, later becoming white and shining, and known as the *lineæ albicantes*. The breasts are full and knotty, and often exude a watery milk. The external genitalia are swollen, the vagina is capacious, the os uteri is low down, and the muco-sanguineous discharge from the uterus, known as the *lochia*, and characterized by its peculiar odor, is usually present. No one of these signs can be relied upon as proof that a woman has recently been delivered; but, if they all be present together, they would constitute a very strong presumption of it. Should the woman have died shortly after delivery, not only would the signs just mentioned be present, but in addition the uterus would be found enlarged, measuring between nine and ten inches in length, its cavity lined with remains of the decidua, and the point of attachment of the placenta marked by a gangrenous-looking spot. In all cases of infanticide, the mother not only endeavors to conceal the fact that she has given birth to a child, but more especially to conceal the body of the child. The concealment of pregnancy is not an offense in the eye of the law; but the concealment of a birth, constituting a misdemeanor, renders the woman committing it liable to punishment. As the woman, however, who is convicted upon this charge is punished upon the ground of having concealed the body of the dead infant rather than upon that of having concealed its delivery, she makes every effort to get rid of the child.

Means of Committing Infanticide.—Among the different means made use of to destroy the new-born child may be mentioned suffocation, immersion in privies, strangulation, drowning, fracturing of the skull, burning, neglect, wounds, hemorrhage of the navel, exposure to cold, and poisoning.   In fully four-fifths of cases of infanticide death is due to asphyxia in one form or another. Statistics show that 50 per cent. of infants criminally destroyed are suffocated, 12 per cent. immersed in privies, 10 per cent. strangled, and 5 per cent. drowned.*   Infants are also not infrequently destroyed by fractures of the skull and by neglect.   Death caused by burns, wounds, hemorrhage of the navel, and exposure to cold occurs less often, however, in cases of infanticide, and in frequency in about the order mentioned.

* Tardieu: " Etude Médico-legale sur l'Infanticide," Paris, 1868, p. 99.

CHAPTER XIII.

Identity of the Living—Feigned Bodily Diseases—Hypnotism—
Life Insurance—Medical Malpractice—Medical Registration.

Identity of the Living.—In cases involving the inheritance of property, as in the celebrated Tichborne case, medical testimony is occasionally taken in identifying a certain individual as the rightful heir. Similarly, in cases of assault or of robbery, the assailant must be identified. Thus, in the case where Grimaldi, the celebrated London clown, was asked if he could identify the prisoner in the dock as the person who had robbed him on the highway, he replied that he was unable to do so positively, placing his hand at the same time, however, with one finger turned down in such a position that the prisoner alone saw it, who became instantly deadly pale. The prisoner, for want of evidence, was discharged. For many years afterward, on the occasion of Grimaldi's annual benefit at the old Drury Lane Theater, a stranger presented a ten-pound note at the box office, and this occurred so invariably that Grimaldi asked the ticket agent if he had ever noticed anything peculiar about the stranger. The agent answered he had *lost a finger on one of his hands*.

It might naturally be supposed that the identity of a person could be satisfactorily established by the family of which the person claimed to be a member. Yet there have occurred cases in which a whole family have been made to believe by an impostor that he was the husband, brother, son, long since supposed to have perished at sea, killed in battle, etc. Thus, some centuries ago (1539), one Arnauld de Tilh, after having made himself perfectly familiar with the past life of his comrade in arms, Martin Guerre, and obtained some of his personal effects, went to Toulouse, the home of Guerre, and personated the latter so perfectly that he was accepted as such by the wife, sisters, uncle, relatives, and friends of the real Martin, who had left his home eight years previously, enlisted in the army, lost a leg in battle in Flanders, whereby he was there detained. After some years, however, the suspicions of the uncle were aroused as to Arnauld de Tilh being really his nephew Martin Guerre, and he had Arnauld arrested; but the evidence submitted at the two trials was so conflicting in character that the impostor would have probably escaped exposure had not the real Martin Guerre returned on a wooden leg, unexpectedly, from Flanders, to his home in Toulouse. It was not until that moment that the wife and sisters of Martin Guerre admitted that they had been imposed upon by de Tilh, and at once implored pardon of Martin for the wrong and injuries they had done him. The impostor, Arnauld de Tilh, was sentenced to be burnt, and before execution confessed his crime.

In cases like that just mentioned and the Tichborne case medical testimony will be required to establish satisfactorily the identity of the claimant. In this connection it may be stated, therefore, that among the more important means of identification may be mentioned the size of the person, the shape and size of the nose, eyes (Figs. 41, 42, 43), ears, foot-prints, the dress, kind of voice, the presence of moles, scars, deformities, nævi, tattoo marks, etc. It is an important and well-established fact that scars due to either injuries or wounds, when the true skin has been involved, are never effaced. In recent years a most

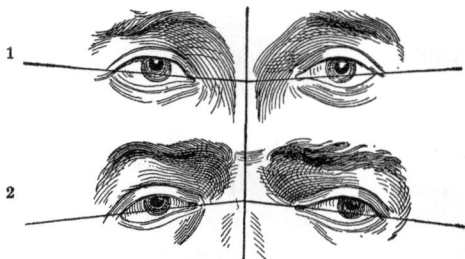

Fig. 41.—1, Photograph of eyes of Roger Tichborne; 2, of Arthur Orton, the claimant.

admirable system, that of Bertillon, based upon photographs, measurement of the eyes, nose (Figs. 41, 42, 43), etc., has been adopted by the French government, and to

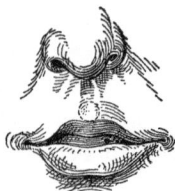

Fig. 42.—Photograph of nose, etc., of Arthur Orton.

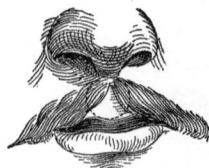

Fig. 43.—Photograph of nose, etc., of Roger Tichborne.

some extent elsewhere, as a means of identifying, more particularly criminals.

In relation to the subject of personal identity, a few words with reference to the distance at which persons can be seen and sounds heard do not appear inappropriate.

A man of ordinary height may be seen on a clear day and on level ground at a distance of from two to three miles, though not necessarily recognized. The recognition of a person depends not only upon being seen, but upon the appreciation of the peculiarities afforded by his size, gait, complexion, color of hair and eyes, etc. Even the best known persons are not always recognized at a distance of one hundred and nine yards; less well-known ones not being recognized even though but thirty yards away. Well-known persons cannot be recognized in the clearest moonlight twenty yards away, and by starlight at a distance exceeding twelve feet, though the light from a flash of lightning or from a pistol-shot may enable a person to recognize another as a thief or an assailant.* Thus, in a well-known instance a lady returning from India by sea was awakened on a dark night in her cabin by a noise, which a sudden flash of lightning enabled her to see was due to a man ransacking her trunk, and further to see him so distinctly as to be able to identify him the next morning. Some of the stolen articles being found upon the man, the latter confessed having committed the theft.

Again, in the case of one Haines, indicted for shooting at three Bow Street officers on the highway, one of the latter deposed that he could distinctly see by the flash of the pistol that the man at the chaise door rode a horse of such peculiar shape that he could pick it out from among fifty horses (which as a matter of fact he did readily recognize), and that the man riding the horse wore a rough shag brown greatcoat.† On the other

* Woodman and Tidy: *op. cit.,* pp. 639–641.
† Guy and Ferrier: *op. cit.,* p. 25.

hand, Professor Gineau deposed at the trial of the supposed assailant of the Sieur Labbe, that his experiments proved that the light emitted by the firing of primings, though strong, was so transient that "it was scarcely possible to see distinctly the form of a head, and that of the face could not be recognized."

The distance at which sounds can be heard, such as the report of a gun or a pistol, being dependent upon the condition of the atmosphere, moisture, direction of the wind, is too variable to be positively stated. As is well known, however, the velocity of sound being at mean temperature about 1130 feet in a second, if a flash of light is seen and a report is heard afterward, on the supposition that they were simultaneously produced, the distance separating the person who fired and the one hearing the report can be calculated.

Feigned bodily diseases very frequently demand the attention of the medical examiner, especially in the cases of soldiers, sailors, and prisoners, who resort to any and every pretext to shirk their duties; and of civilians, who hope in this way to avoid serving on juries, appearing as witnesses, or to escape military service. It is almost incredible what malingerers will resort to in order to accomplish their purpose, indulging in the most disgusting performances: swallowing feces, urine, blood, mutilating themselves, as occasion may require. Disease is sometimes simulated by simply lying, or by mimicry, or cunning; at other times by the aid of trusses, splints, bandages, spectacles, crutches, and such means. The motives inducing a person to simulate disease are usually fear, gain, laziness, notoriety. Thus, for example, it is not unusual, especially abroad, where military service is compulsory for such as are liable, to cut off a finger, break a tooth, or put out an eye, to avoid conscription. The hope of gain is a very common motive, as in the attempts so often made to obtain damages for injuries incurred in railroad accidents. Beggars and others, to escape work and to get into hospitals or almshouses, often feign disease.

Hysterical persons, especially women, will stoop to every kind of deceit, and submit even to harsh treatment, through a pure love of notoriety. While there is no kind of disease or injury which malingerers will not simulate in order to accomplish their purpose, whatever that may be, among the most common of these may be mentioned the feigning of fever, heart disease, consumption, hæmaturia, incontinence of urine, epilepsy, paralysis, catalepsy, deafness, dumbness, blindness, tumors, wounds, etc. Malingerers appear to have been as common in ancient as in modern times. Even so far back as the time of Galen rules were given for the guidance of the physician in detecting such frauds.* All such cases of malingering demand the greatest patience and tact on the part of the medical examiner. Not only one, but several visits may be required before the examiner can be satisfied that the case is one of malingering. The visits should be paid at an hour when the suspected person is least likely to expect them. The parts of the body said to be diseased or injured should be examined unclothed, thoroughly exposed, all dressings and bandages being removed. No attention or importance should be attached to the statements of either the person supposed to be malingering or his relatives or friends. The prescribing of some disagreeable medicine, or the suggestion

* "London Medical Gazette," vol. xvii, p. 989.

of using anæsthetics, and performing a dangerous operation, may sometimes frighten the individual into confessing imposture.* In some obstinate cases, however, all means, even of a severe character, fail to elicit confession.

Relation of Hypnotism to Crime.—The question of the possibility of a crime being committed by an individual when hypnotized, at the suggestion of another, and the responsibility so incurred by one or both, is still under discussion. It is true that experiments have been made which show the remote possibility of crime being committed under such circumstances, as in the case, for example, of a hypnotized woman plunging a dirk into a manikin dressed as a woman, at the command of another. Nevertheless, according to most medical jurists, there is no evidence whatever that a murder has ever been committed in this way.† In hypnotized persons, women especially, hysteria constitutes so important a factor, and hysteria is so often simulated, that it would become difficult, if not impossible, for the medical examiner to state positively to what extent a person committing murder or any other crime when hypnotized should be held responsible.

* Zacchias: *op. cit.*, Lib. iii, Tit. ii, Quaest. ii, p. 288.

† It should be mentioned that, according to the daily papers, a murder having been committed at Winfield, Kansas, May 5, 1894, by a man when hypnotized, the Supreme Court of that State sustained the ruling of the lower county court, which had convicted the hypnotizer of murder, but adjudged the hypnotized, who had actually committed the murder, innocent. If such a verdict was ever actually rendered, it is the first case, so far as known to the author, in which hypnotism has been held *in foro* as a sufficient ground for the acquittal of a person charged with murder.

Life Insurance.—A life insurance may be regarded as a contract, the deed being termed a policy, whereby a company, in consideration of a premium paid in installments or in a lump sum, agrees to pay a definite sum to the heirs of the insured at death, or to the insured at some definite period of life. In the case of the former, the amount insured for being payable only at death, it becomes incumbent upon the heirs to prove most positively, and to the entire satisfaction of the company, that the insured person is actually dead. For example, in cases of persons who have disappeared, who went to sea and were never heard of again, questions as to presumption of death or of survivorship may demand the attention of the medical examiner. The question as to the general health of an applicant for a policy of insurance—the tendency to disease through inheritance, alcoholism, excessive use of tobacco, or other causes—is that which brings the medical profession in the most intimate relation with the insurance companies. In almost all the lawsuits in contested life insurance policies, the points contested are with reference to what was actually meant by certain medical terms, such as diseases, habits tending to shorten life, etc.

It is astonishing what a difference of opinion prevails among even intelligent people as to what constitutes a temperate person, many an individual who takes several drinks of brandy or whisky a day considering himself perfectly temperate, and so stating to the medical examiner, utterly unconscious of his health being gradually undermined, and of his life being shortened by the daily use of alcohol. It is due to such a difference of opinion as to the effect of alcohol upon the system that the question of intemperance has given rise to so much discussion in cases of life insurance. While it is undoubtedly true that there have been exceptional instances of individuals enjoying good health and living to a good old age who had been in the habit of drinking, and more particularly whisky, all their lives, nevertheless it cannot be denied that, as a general rule, the habitual use of alcohol, in perverting nutrition, induces diseases of the heart, liver, and kidneys, and so tends to shorten life. It should be mentioned, however, that if the habits of the individual at the time of insurance were temperate, the fact that intemperance was subsequently developed would not debar the heirs from recovery upon the policy.

What has just been said of the use of alcohol with reference to the shortening of life applies equally to the influence of the morphia habit. The concealment of the fact that an applicant for a policy of life insurance was an opium eater at the time of the application would justify the company in refusing to pay the heirs the insurance.

There is no doubt that insanity also tends to shorten life, and, with the view of avoiding future complications which might arise upon this point, every insurance policy should contain a direct question on insanity, the insurance company reserving to itself the privilege of insuring or not, according to the particular circumstances of the case.

Litigation in cases of life insurance not infrequently arises in consequence of the insured person committing suicide after the taking out of the policy. Under such circumstances a company would certainly be justified in refusing to pay the insurance if it could be proved that the suicide was committed with the intention of paying off debts or leaving money to the heirs. If, however, the suicide was due to insanity, clearly developed after the policy had been taken out, the heirs would undoubtedly be entitled to the payment of the insurance.

From what has just been said of the relationship of the alcohol and opium habit, insanity, suicide, to life insurance, it is obvious that, for the interest of the company, as well as for that of the insured, a most thorough examination should be made as to the health of the individual at the time of the application for the policy. Not only should all the printed questions of the policy be satisfactorily answered by the applicant, but the latter should be most carefully questioned orally by the medical examiner of the company. It is the concealment of the true state of the health of the applicant, either fraudulently or unintentionally, at the time that the policy was taken out, which gives rise to most of the lawsuits in cases of life insurance.

In insurance cases death is not infrequently simulated in order to deceive the company. Thus, in 1874 a man named Goss, whose life had been insured, conspired with his wife and one Udderzook to get the insurance company to pay the insurance to the wife. It was represented to the company that Goss had been burnt to death in a wooden house where he had been in the habit of working, and the charred remains of a dead body that had been put in the house before it was set on fire were offered as proof of Goss's death. Goss in the mean time disguised himself and went to New York, where he soon tired of the kind of life he was obliged to live to avoid discovery, and threatened to betray Udderzook. The latter then decoyed Goss to come to West Chester, Pennsylvania, where he murdered him, for which Udderzook was tried, convicted, and hanged.

It is well known, also, that in many instances persons
14

have been murdered on account of the insurance upon their lives. Thus, for example, during the years 1855–1856 Ann Palmer, Walter Palmer, and J. P. Cook were all poisoned by William Palmer, to enable the latter to obtain from the companies the large amounts for which their lives had been insured. Had not suspicion been aroused and Palmer arrested, tried, and executed, two other persons would undoubtedly have been murdered by Palmer for the same object.*

It is stated that the defendant, a woman, in R. *v.* Cotten (Durham Lent Assizes, 1873), who was executed for poisoning her stepson with arsenic, had murdered no less than twenty different persons, all of whose lives she had insured in different offices.

Another well-known case is that of Dr. de la Pommerais, who, after having insured the life of a woman named Pauw, poisoned her with digitalin.†

Some years ago the author was called upon to make a post-mortem examination upon the body of a man named Armstrong, who had evidently been murdered. It was subsequently shown that the life of the deceased had been insured in favor of one Hunter, who was tried and convicted of having murdered Armstrong for the insurance, for which crime he was hanged in Camden, N. J.

Numerous other cases might be mentioned which have occurred in recent years, showing how prevalent is the crime of murder for the purpose of procuring insurance money. Physicians should be most careful, therefore, in giving

* Taylor: "Medical Jurisprudence," seventh American edition. p. 867.

† Wharton and Stillé : *op. cit.,* vol. III, p. 805.

death-certificates in cases of insurance policies, the latter being so often effected in a most lax way.

Medical Malpractice.—Actions for damages for large amounts are so often brought against physicians on the charge of malpractice, that it is well for the medical profession to realize that the law affords, even to the most distinguished of its members, under such circumstances, no especial protection. In order, therefore, to avoid the annoyance and loss of time always entailed by such suits, howsoever they may terminate, it is most important that practitioners should never guarantee or contract to effect a cure, even in the simplest kind of cases. Whatever the nature of the difficulties arising in the case may have been, however improbable that they should have occurred, or that they could have been foreseen, is immaterial, the law not accepting any such excuses for the failure on the part of the practitioner to fulfil his contract to cure.

Such being the case, how unwise would it be for a surgeon to promise that he will cure a deformity, or for the gynæcologist to guarantee the safe removal of an abdominal tumor when there is always a risk that death may follow any serious operation! All that a practitioner can be expected to say is that he will do the best he can for his patient. The law only demands that he will exhibit in the practice of his profession a fair and competent degree of skill. It must be admitted, however, that it becomes difficult, if not impossible, to say, under certain circumstances, just what constitutes legally a reasonable or ordinary amount of professional skill. It is evident that the skill indispensable to the success of a physician or surgeon practising in a metropolis must be far greater than that demanded of one practising in a village. The legal term *ordinary skill* is, therefore, far from being a definite one, and from the very nature of the case must have a varied application. Not only ordinary skill, such as is demanded in the successful performance of a surgical operation, must be exhibited, but ordinary care and attention in the after-treatment must be paid the patient as well. The bandaging, the dressings, the diet, must be all carefully looked after, as neglect of the same, involving possibly the occurrence of secondary hemorrhage, mortification, pyæmia, or even only deformity, will render the practitioner justly liable to a suit for damages.

On the other hand, a practitioner should not be held responsible for not prescribing some particular remedy or for the failure of some one remedy to cure, since the greatest difference of opinion prevails among therapeutists as to the efficacy of all so-called "remedies." It is still a question among medical jurists whether a practitioner renders himself liable to prosecution in deviating somewhat from the usual manner of performing an operation, as, for example, in vaccinating on some part of the arm other than the part usually selected for that purpose. As a matter of fact, it may be mentioned, however, that in one instance in which the virus was introduced nearer to the elbow than usual and serious inflammation followed, the court ruled that the attending physician was responsible for all the bad consequences attending the case.

As the law recognizes no particular school of medicine, all doctors have about the same standing legally. Every practitioner is supposed, however, to practise according to the system of medicine taught in the school of which he is a graduate. It might be supposed, therefore, that if a violent remedy was administered or a surgical operation performed, by an individual who had received no medical education whatever, in the event of serious consequences, death ensuing, the law would hold such a person criminally responsible. But, strange to say, there have been cases, as, for example, when a prolapsed uterus, being mistaken for a placenta, was torn out by a midwife and a fatal hemorrhage ensued; and yet the Chief Justice of England, Lord Ellenborough, ruled that there was not sufficient evidence to convict the prisoner of the crime of murder, and the defendant was acquitted.

Suits brought against physicians for malpractice are usually for damages—civil rather than criminal in character. By far the greater number of such cases are purely for the purpose of blackmail, the plaintiff usually securing the services of counsel with the understanding that if he wins the suit his fee will be part of the damages awarded. Among such cases may be mentioned those in which a shortening of a limb, the stiffness of a joint, a certain deformity, are alleged as having been due to the neglect of the surgeon in the treatment of a fracture or of a dislocation. In all such cases it is incumbent upon the plaintiff to prove that the alleged injury or disease was due to the attending surgeon, and that the same might have been foreseen and avoided by proper treatment. Malpractice can only be proved when it is shown that the practitioner has set aside established principles and neglected to make use of means universally held by the profession to be necessary in a given case. It must be shown, however, that in all probability the treatment according to such established principles would accomplish the desired end, that such treatment never proves detrimental, and that it is sanctioned by the general practice of the profession.

It should be mentioned in this connection that gratuitousness will not exempt a practitioner from a charge of malpractice if it can be proved that his treatment was improper, or that he neglected the patient. On the other hand, a patient who refuses to co-operate with his physician cannot recover damages for any injury so sustained, unless the latter can be shown to have been due to malpractice. As it has been decided that a physician who takes with him, to a confinement case, any one except a physician or a student of medicine, renders himself liable for damages, except in cases of necessity, it would be well under any circumstances for him to obtain the consent of the patient before introducing a stranger into the sickroom.

In connection with the general subject of medical malpractice it may be mentioned that apothecaries render themselves liable to suits for damages or even to criminal prosecution, if it can be shown that, through their ignorance or carelessness, or that of inexperienced clerks in the putting up and selling of medicines, serious or fatal consequences ensued.

Medical Registration.—According to law every physician must register, and, for the benefit of young physicians just beginning the practice of their profession, the full text of the registration law is here given: "It shall be the duty of every practising physician and of every practitioner of midwifery, on or before the first day of July next ensuing (the day on which the law goes into effect), to report his, her, or their names and places of residence to the health officer at the office of the board of health, and it shall be the duty of the health officer to have the same properly registered in index form in suitable books. In the event

of any of the persons specified removing to any other place
of residence, it shall be their duty to notify the health officer
of the fact within thirty days after such removal, except
where the persons removing shall cease to act in such official capacity as makes them subject to the provisions of
this act".

PART II.

INSANITY.

PART II.

INSANITY.

Classification of Varieties of Insanity—Idiocy—Mania—Dementia—Medico-legal Relations of Insanity—Criminal Responsibility
—Medico-legal Terms in Insanity—Feigned Mental Diseases.

THE subject of insanity has so extensive a range as
to render it impossible, within the limits of this work,
to do more than indicate its salient features, more especially from a medico-legal point of view. Every practi-

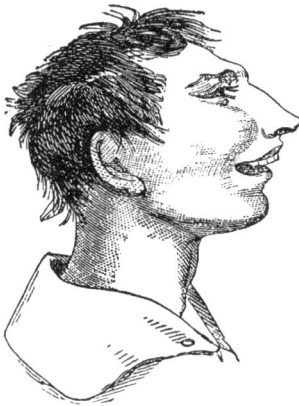

Fig. 44.—Idiocy (Ferrier).　　　Fig. 45.—Epileptic mania (Ferrier).

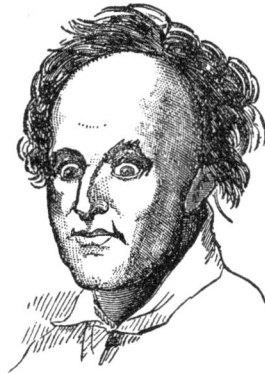

tioner should appreciate the importance of the fact that
at any moment he may be called upon to visit a person
said to have lost his reason, and should be qualified,
therefore, to express an opinion as to his sanity.

Varieties of Insanity.—Systematic writers upon the subject of insanity differ very much in the manner in which they classify the different varieties of insanity. For our present purpose insanity may be conveniently regarded as being of three kinds—Idiocy or Amentia, Mania, and Dementia* or Want of Mind, Disordered Mind, and Loss of Mind.

Insanity:

- Amentia
  - Imbecility
  - Idiocy
- Mania
  - Mania Proper
  - Melancholia
  - Partial Intellectual
  - Moral
  - Partial Moral
    - Kleptomania
    - Pyromania
    - Dipsomania
    - Homicidal
    - Suicidal
    - Puerperal
- Dementia—Paralytic (Paresis)

Idiocy.—*Dementia naturalis*, or idiocy, differs from all other kinds of mental disease in being congenital, depending upon an arrest of cerebral development. There are various degrees of it, varying from a condition in which there is an entire absence of mind to one in which there is a glimmering of intelligence, as in imbecility. Imbeciles are usually docile, and, in some instances, can be taught, by careful management, to talk and even to read. The causes of idiocy are usually syphilis, intemperance (of the parents), consanguineous marriages.

* Ray, I. : " A Treatise on the Medical Jurisprudence of Insanity," fifth edition, 1871, pp. 84, 430, 577; Georget : " De la Folie," Paris, 1820, p. 101; Mandsley, M. D. : " Physiology and Pathology of the Mind," London, 1868, p. 253.

Idiots (Fig. 44) can generally be recognized by the small size of the head (except in the case of congenital hydrocephalus, in which the head is very large), thickness of the lips, enlargement of the tongue, salivary glands, and tonsils, vaulting of the hard palate, irregularity of the teeth, with tendency to decay, deficiency of the lobules of the ear, defective vision, weakness in the fingers and thumbs. Idiocy is frequently associated with goiter, or enlargement of the thyroid gland, the condition being known as cretinism. Idiots are not only characterized by the absence or deficiency of intellectual power, but also by undue development of the animal part of their nature, as shown by their filthy habits, gluttony, etc. Upon post-mortem examination, the convolutions and fissures in the brain of an idiot are usually found less numerous and less complicated in their arrangement than in the brain of an intelligent person. Together with the deficiency of the gray matter of the cortex, due to so simple a type of brain, important parts of the latter, such as basal ganglia, corpus callosum, cerebellum, may be undeveloped or even entirely absent. Neither idiocy nor imbecility is likely to be mistaken for mania, for, although the intelligence in the latter conditions is perverted and irregular, hallucinations being common, there is not that entire absence of it which is so characteristic of idiocy. However, as we shall see presently, idiocy, in some respects, resembles dementia. It need hardly be added that idiots are entirely irresponsible, both from a civil and a criminal point of view.

Mania (Fig. 45) is understood as a general perversion of the mental faculties, accompanied usually with more or less excitement, which in certain cases may amount even to fury. The reasoning powers are not absolutely lost, but are rather confused, disturbed, disordered. There is no orderly sequence of thoughts; ideas follow each other without any relationship. At one moment the maniac may be tractable, pious in his expressions, singing hymns; at another, ungovernable, abusive, blasphemous. He sings, dances, laughs, then cries, tears off his clothes, breaks anything that he can lay his hands on, often at such times exhibiting great strength. The skin is dry and hot; the eye has a very characteristic expression— a fixed, wild, brilliant sort of stare. The pulse and respiration are usually quick and the temperature high. The appetite is generally voracious. The urine and feces are often voided involuntarily. Sexual desire—erotomania— is usually increased, and when so occurring in women is known as *nymphomania;* in men, as *satyriasis.*

One of the most striking features of mania is the total alteration wrought in the feelings of one so affected toward the members of his family; the maniac becoming suspicious of and hating those whom he had formerly naturally loved. When haunted by delusions, which is not infrequently the case, he may become so dangerous as to necessitate physical restraint. Systematic writers upon the subject of insanity consider mania to be of different kinds, distinguishing the varieties, as mania proper or intellectual mania, which we have just described, melancholia, partial intellectual mania, moral mania, partial moral mania, the latter being manifested more particularly as kleptomania, pyromania, dipsomania, and homicidal, suicidal, puerperal mania. But, whatever views may be held by systematists concerning different kinds of insanity, moral, emotional, intellectual, etc., it should be under-

stood that the law recognizes only one kind of insanity—
that which affects the mind, the latter being adjudged
as unsound when affected with delusions that cannot be
dispelled.

Melancholia may be regarded as a variety of mania,
differing more especially from the latter in being characterized by depression rather than excitement, by the
patient refusing food rather than partaking of it eagerly.
The face is pale and pinched, the eyelids droop, the pupils
are dilated. The patient sits for hours at a time doing
nothing, brooding over melancholy thoughts; he is often
of a religious nature, suspicious of being persecuted,
burned, poisoned, etc.; often dirty in habits, soiling his
clothes and linen, utterly indifferent to his personal
appearance.

Partial intellectual mania is characterized by the fact
that a person who suffers from this form of mental disease
is possessed of some one notion contrary to his own experience, as well as to all common sense. He may imagine
that his legs are made of glass, or his stomach is full of
lizards and snakes; or, if the individual be a woman,
that she is pregnant by the devil.* Persons afflicted
with this form of mania, but apparently sensible enough
in other respects, have imagined themselves to be the
Pope, President of the United States, etc. This form
of mania is often called monomania, it being supposed
that the mind is only deranged on one subject, the insanity restricted to one delusion, the remaining faculties
being unimpaired by disease. It is very difficult to
believe, however, if not impossible, that such a mental
condition can exist; that a brain could be so diseased

* Ray: *op. cit.*, p. 200.

in an individual as to give rise to a well-marked form
of mania and yet at the same time leave the remaining
faculties unaffected in all other respects. The term monomania has lost, therefore, much of its significance in
recent years, and is fast becoming an obsolete term in
the literature of insanity.

General Moral Mania.—This form of mania supposes
that a morbid perversion of the natural affections, temper,
and habits of an individual can exist without any noticeable
derangement of the intellect. As such a doctrine is not
sustained by the decisions of the courts, and is incom-
patible with the principles of penal jurisprudence and
psychology,* it is not necessary for us to dwell further
upon it than merely to say that the plea of so-called
moral mania will not be regarded by law as excusing
or palliating crime.

It need hardly be added that if insanity of the moral
system cannot coexist with the sanity of the mental,—
that is, if there can be no moral mania in general,—there
can be then no partial moral mania in particular. The
various kinds of mania referred to under the latter head
are to be regarded, therefore, in every case o be due
to some kind of aberration of the intellect, and further,
that they are not monomanias in the sense in which that
word is ordinarily used, there being no such form of
insanity as real monomania.

Kleptomania, or the disposition to steal, is exhibited
so often by persons in good circumstances that this pecu-
liarity cannot be attributed to want, but to some aberration of the intellect. In all trials of kleptomaniacs, it
must be proved that the defendant is incapable of appre-

* Wharton and Stillé: *op. cit.*, vol. i, p. 432

ciating what constitutes the crime of theft; otherwise the plea of this form of insanity would be the favorite defense of all professional thieves.

Pyromania, or the insane desire to set fire to anything,—barns, dwelling-houses, churches,—is a less common form of mania than kleptomania. It appears to be often associated with epileptic insanity. As instances of pyromania may be mentioned the case of Jonathan Martin, who imagined he was deputed by God to burn down the Cathedral of York. Another well-known case is that of Maria Frank, an illiterate peasant in whom a few coppers' worth of spirit developed an irresistible impulse to set houses on fire. In the case of James Gibson, tried before the High Court of Justiciary, Edinburgh (1844), for firing certain premises, it was held by the defense that the state of the man's mind was such as to render him irresponsible for the act. Notwithstanding that the medical evidence favored the plea of insanity, the jury negatived the latter, and the prisoner was sentenced to transportation for fourteen years.*

Dipsomania, or the craving for drink, differs from the desire for liquor shown by those who indulge daily in the use of alcohol in the circumstance that it is followed by long remissions in the thirst for it. During these periods there is not only no desire, but often a loathing, for it. With the return of the craving, the individual will literally soak himself with spirits for days and weeks at a time, often secluding himself and shunning society of all kinds.

In this connection, the criminal responsibility of drunkards may be as appropriately considered here as else-

* Wharton and Stillé: *op. cit.*, vol. i, p. 495.

where. It is certainly a strange anomaly that while the unsoundness of mind due to excessive intoxication will disqualify, according to law, an individual from signing a will or making a contract, nevertheless, should such an individual violate in any way the criminal law, he will be held responsible and punished accordingly. It should be mentioned, however, that while drunkenness is not regarded by law as an excuse for crime, the unsoundness of mind, amounting in many cases to insanity, induced by excessive intoxication or the prolonged use of ardent spirits must be taken into consideration and ought to palliate, if not to excuse. Undoubtedly, irresponsibility would be inferred by the law in the case of a person whose mind had been weakened by habitual drinking unless it could be shown that, at the moment of the commission of the crime, the individual was fully conscious of the nature of the deed.

A murder committed by a drunken man would not be excused, however, by the law if he had voluntarily become drunk before perpetrating the crime. In all such trials, an extenuating circumstance would be the fact that the defendant had no grudge or malice against the deceased, the absence of any motive to murder, malice aforethought, but had committed the murder when under the influence of drink. In many murder trials, however, where insanity superinduced by intoxication is alleged as the defense, the court not infrequently finds it difficult to decide whether the defendant committed the murder when drunk or whether he got drunk to commit the murder.

It is obvious, therefore, that the safety of the community demands that the greatest caution should be exercised by the law in admitting that drunkenness is an excuse for murder. Few persons indeed have the nerve to deliberately commit murder without fortifying themselves with liquor or stimulus of some kind, and if it were generally understood that drunkenness renders an individual irresponsible, every individual intending to commit murder would get drunk first in order to escape the penalty of the crime, and it would be impossible then to ever convict any one of homicide.

It may be mentioned, in connection with the responsibility of drunkards, that somnambulists cannot be held responsible for their acts, for, in such a condition as that of somnambulism, there can be, from the very nature of the case, no motives to commit crime, the intellect being in abeyance.

Homicidal Mania.—This form of mania may be associated with irrational motives, delusions, or without any motive whatever, the desire to kill arising instantaneously and apparently uncontrollably, irresistibly. The question to be decided by the court in such cases is whether the homicidal impulse is really irresistible or can be resisted. In the former case the act is involuntary, beyond control, and the defendant should, therefore, be adjudged insane and acquitted of murder. In the second case the action is a voluntary one and the defendant is responsible and should be convicted of murder.

In instances of this kind of insanity, it will be generally learned, from the previous history of the case, that the individual had been injured at some previous period, as by a fall upon the head, in consequence of which he had become more or less morose and melancholic at times. The maniac may murder a number of persons at once, the victims, not infrequently, being members of his own family, to whom he had been previously devotedly attached, and without any motive whatever. Further, the maniac makes no effort to escape from the consequences of his act, as an ordinary sane murderer would do. He may even boast of what he has done, saying that he had been directly inspired to do what he did.

The plea of homicidal mania,—the irresistible desire to murder,—like that of drunkenness, has so often, however, been improperly alleged as a defense for murder, that it has given rise in many cases, in the mind of the prosecution, to an irresistible desire to hang, and hang it did.

Suicidal Mania.—While, in most cases of suicide, the verdict of the coroner's jury—the latter actuated, no doubt, by kindly feelings for the family of the deceased—is death by his or her hands while laboring under temporary insanity, there can be no doubt that perfectly sane persons commit suicide. In ancient times it was a common custom for persons who were at war to take their own lives rather than take the chances of falling into the hands of their conquerors and run the risk of torture and death. It is a matter of everyday occurrence for men who have failed in business to commit suicide rather than to face their creditors, disaster, and financial ruin. Indeed, so many suicides are committed, not only intentionally, but intelligently, that it becomes very often difficult to say that the self-destruction was due to insanity. The disposition to commit suicide is, in many instances, undoubtedly inherited, inasmuch as it is well known that the members of certain families for generations have been in the habit of taking their own lives. A remarkable feature in suicide is the regularity with which it occurs, and the frequency with which it is committed in the same way. Indeed, under certain circumstances, the perpetration of the act and the uniformity of the means by which it is accomplished may not inappropriately be said to be epidemic.*

Puerperal insanity, which is one of the most distressing kinds of mania, attacks women after delivery, within a period varying from a few days to several weeks. It occurs usually before the stoppage of the lochia; albumin appears in the urine, and the flow of milk is suppressed. A woman suffering from this form of mania may be either foul-mouthed or taciturn and pious in her talk, and may often be troubled with religious delusions. She may either totally neglect her infant, or take such a dislike to it that she sooner or later destroys it, and frequently in the most horrible manner. It should be remembered, therefore, by the medical jurist, that, in certain cases of infanticide, the mother may have been afflicted with puerperal insanity, and that under such circumstances she should not be held responsible for the consequences of her actions.

Dementia, or fatuity, beginning with a simple enfeeblement of the intellect, terminates with an entire extinction of the mental powers. This form of disease is characterized by absence of ideas, accompanied by depression, rather than, as is mania, by exaggerated mental activity, with excitement. It may follow acute mania or melancholia; is often due to disease of the brain, the result of injury, and is frequently incidental to old age. The

* Buckle: "History of Civilization in England," chap. i, p. 25; Morselli, H.: "Suicide: An Essay on Comparative Moral Statistics," New York, 1882.

countenance in dementia (Fig. 46) is pale, and the expression is a peculiarly vacant one. A most striking feature is loss of memory, the patient, in an advanced stage of the disease, forgetting even what has transpired within a moment or two. Individuals affected with this disease act in an undecided, silly, childish manner, repeating themselves in conversation, appearing neither to like nor dislike their former friends and associates, moving about in an aimless, listless way. A disposition is often exhibited in this disease to hoard up articles of no value.

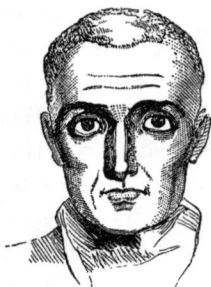

Fig. 46.—Dementia (paresis) (Ferrier).

Paralytic dementia, also known as general paralysis or paresis of the insane, appears to be due more especially to disease of the gray matter of the convolutions of the brain. This form of disease may be caused by syphilis, alcoholism, excessive mental work. The first symptoms of general paresis of the insane are a certain fretfulness, irritability of manner, accompanied by carelessness in dress, etc. The patient becomes deluded with the idea of being possessed of great wealth or great physical strength. As the disease advances, the muscular power becomes much weakened, and the gait unsteady. The tongue trembles when protruded, the lips are tremulous, and difficulty is experienced in pronouncing certain words. Vision becomes affected. A bloody, gelatinous swelling of the ear develops, the so-called "hæmatoma auris," the contents of which, resembling the extravasations under the dura mater in pachymeningitis, appear to be due to a degeneration of the branches of the carotid artery.   The prognosis in general paresis of the insane is always unfavorable, death taking place within a period varying from two to ten years.

Medico-legal Relations of Insanity.—Having described, in a general way at least, the most important forms of mental disease, it remains now to consider them in their medico-legal relations.   Should a person be determined to be insane, the first question to be considered is as to the degree of the insanity, and more especially as to the civil and criminal responsibility of the individual. As out of this twofold inquiry arise all medico-legal questions of insanity, there should be no misunderstanding as to what is meant by civil and criminal responsibility. Civil responsibility implies the capability of managing one's own business, taking an intelligent part in the ordinary affairs of civil life, making contracts, wills, etc. Criminal responsibility renders the perpetrator of any crime, such as theft, arson, murder, liable to punishment, supposing the person sufficiently sane at the time of the commission of the deed to be held responsible.   In all cases of insanity the practitioner who assumes the responsibility of giving advice should have had a great deal of experience in treating insanity, and should exercise great caution before he advises that a person should be deprived of his liberty and placed under restraint.   Before positively expressing the opinion that the patient is insane, and setting forth the facts upon which such an opinion is based, the physician should satisfy himself, beyond doubt, that the person alleged to be insane is really so.   Not only one visit, but several visits may have to be made before all doubts as to the insanity of the patient are removed.   In case the practitioner advises that the patient be treated at home, it should be distinctly understood that he is relieved of all responsibility for the restraint, that being assumed by the friends or the members of the family. The form of certificate by which an insane person can be removed to an asylum is fixed by statute, and no other form is valid in America. In Pennsylvania the certificate must be signed by two respectable physicians, who have practised medicine for five years, both of whom must have examined the patient within one week of their signing the certificate, and who both must testify under oath that it is absolutely necessary for the safety of the individual and the public that the patient shall be placed under restraint in an asylum. The physicians signing the certificate should not be related by blood or marriage, or be officially connected in any way with the asylum in which the patient is to be confined. Practitioners cannot be too cautious in signing a certificate for the placing of a patient in an insane asylum, false commitment rendering them liable to heavy punishment by an action at law. It should be remembered that, in many instances, physicians have been deceived by relatives interested in the management or disposal of an estate, and induced by their misrepresentations of the state of mind of the patient to sign a certificate consigning him or her to an insane asylum.

Judgment and caution must be exercised in signing the discharge of a patient from an asylum by the physician in charge, as well as in signing one of commitment. Patients are usually removed from an asylum by the members of their family or friends at the discretion and with the approval of the superintendent. In America there is no law preventing the liberation of the insane on recovery, except in cases of homicidal lunatics who have been committed to an asylum by an order of the court.

Civil Responsibility of the Insane.—The opinion of the practitioner is occasionally asked as to the capacity of an individual to make a will, to sign a contract, or to marry. It should be remembered, strange as it may appear, that less mental capacity is required by law to make a will than to permit the managing of property or the enjoyment of personal liberty. The courts have ruled in many instances that patients, even when confined in insane asylums, have made good wills, and have held as valid the most absurd wills, it having been shown that such wills were in perfect accordance with the life of the eccentric, but not therefore necessarily insane, testator. In order, however, that a will should be valid, the law requires that the testator should be sane, at least at the time of making the will. A will made when the testator was under the influence of liquor, or narcotized, or afflicted with the delirium of fever, would not be held as valid. A person would not be disqualified, however, from making a will when poisoned by arsenic or strychnia, provided his mind was clear; and the same may be said of a person suffering from typhoid fever, paralysis, or epilepsy. When a physician is consulted as to the capacity of a person to make a will, the examination of the testator should be made in private, or only in the presence of the nurse, or perhaps of one member of the family. The physician should satisfy himself that the testator is not under the influence of liquor, or of any drug; that he fully realizes the importance and the nature of the act he is about to perform; that he is not affected by any delusions; and that no undue influence has been brought to bear upon him.

A most delicate question for the physician to answer, and his advice is often asked upon the subject, is that of the propriety of one person marrying another who has been insane, or in whose family insanity is hereditary. While, as a general rule, all marriages of such a character, as well as those in which there is a tendency in the contracting parties to inherit any disease, are to be discouraged, any advice to the contrary that may be given by the physician will not prevent their taking place, and nothing will be gained by his opposition. The family physician is often called upon to give advice as to the best means of bringing up children begotten by such unfortunate marriages. Hygienic treatment is all that can be recommended in such cases. It ought to be insisted upon, however, that the children should have pure country air, plenty of outdoor exercise, plain but nutritious food; that all excitement, especially at the age of puberty, should be avoided; and, above all, that little or no mental effort should be required, even though the child should thereby grow up comparatively uneducated.

Criminal Responsibility of the Insane.—Of all the questions which the subject of legal medicine gives rise to, there is none more difficult or more worthy of consideration than that of the relations of insanity to criminal responsibility. In nearly every trial for homicide, however brutal or revolting the crime, no matter how outrageous or aggravated the circumstances may be, after every other plea has been urged, the defense, as a last resource, attempts to prove that the murderer was insane. It might be supposed that the sophistry, flimsy rubbish, unworthy of being dignified by the name of argument, advanced by adroit counsel, could speedily be disposed of in all such cases by limiting the discussion to simply determining whether the defendant was afflicted with any mental disorder due to disease. The difficulty, however, which at once arises consists in deciding what shall constitute a test of the existence of a mental disorder. At one time it was universally admitted that an individual was responsible unless totally deprived of his understanding and memory—not knowing what he was doing any more than an infant, brute, or wild beast. The knowledge of right and wrong was later considered as a test of responsibility in criminal cases. The test was afterward so qualified that the knowledge of right and wrong was to have relation only to the particular act of which the individual was accused; and it was still further modified in its being held that the person accused must have a knowledge of the consequences of the act. There can be no doubt, however, that insane persons have not only been fully conscious of the criminality of their acts, but have realized as well their consequences and the punishment to which they rendered themselves liable.

The knowledge of right and wrong, the consciousness of criminality, the realization of liability to punishment being possessed by insane persons, have in recent times led to the claim that only those individuals should be held irresponsible who have lost all power of control over their actions. The test of irresponsibility may be said to be, in this view, then, the proof of a want of will-power, the power of choosing between good and evil being destroyed by disease. The accused would not, however, be held irresponsible if the crime was committed under the influence, temporarily, of liquor, or of a violent burst of passion, the latter condition being often attributed to impulsive or emotional insanity—a form of mental disorder for the existence of which there is no evidence.

Not infrequently medical experts in insanity are also called upon by the courts to state whether a criminal under sentence of death is insane, in order to stay execution.

Medico-legal Terms Defined.—In connection with cases of insanity certain legal terms are frequently made use of rather loosely, such as *illusions, hallucinations, delusions, lucid intervals;* but these terms should be defined, in order that the medical examiner may be qualified to answer intelligently in court questions involving their use. An illusion may be defined as a false impression due to a material basis, the impression being, however, distorted through some defect in the avenue of sense, or of the perceptive center, as in mistaking a tree for a man at night. Hallucinations differ from illusions in being perverted impressions, but without a material basis, at least immediately. A person afflicted with this disorder imagines he hears strange voices, sees people where there are none, etc. Delusions may be defined as beliefs in something purely imaginary, as when a pauper imagines he has become a millionaire, or when a millionaire believes he has lost everything. Should a delusion be so strong as to affect the disposal of an estate by will, as when a parent has come to hate, for no reason, his children, whom he had formerly loved, the capacity to make a will should be disputed. If, however, the delusion with which an individual is affected is not connected in any way with the act about to be performed, the responsibility of such a person would not be questioned. By a lucid interval is meant a temporary intermission of insanity, during which period the individual recovers his reasoning powers. It may last for months, weeks, or only for a few minutes. It not infrequently occurs in mania, and occasionally in dementia, but never in idiocy or imbecility. During a lucid interval the law recognizes the power of a person to sign a contract, to make a will, to exercise civil rights, etc.

Feigned mental diseases are usually considered by writers upon medical jurisprudence separately from feigned bodily disorders. The expression mental disease, whether feigned or not, regarded as something distinct from bodily disease, is, however, an unphilosophical one, as there can be no disease, mental or otherwise, without some underlying change in organization. Whatever may be the psychological views held as to the nature of mind, whether it be regarded as an entity, a something independent—superadded to the body—an almost obsolete view now—or as a function of the nervous system, and, more especially in man, of the cerebral portion of it, a view accepted by all physiologists, is immaterial, at least so far as it affects the view universally accepted that a healthy mind is always found in a healthy body. *Orandum est. ut sit mens sana in corpore sano.*

In connection with the subject of insanity, and as a mere matter of convenience, the subject of feigned mental diseases may be as appropriately considered here as elsewhere. Mental diseases are most frequently feigned by criminals, in the hope of escaping imprisonment or capital punishment. It is frequently very difficult to prove in such cases that the criminal is malingering, insanity in one form or another being so well imitated. The criminal may keep up the deception for months, during which he may rave, beat the door, tear his clothes and bedding, indulge in the foulest language and dirty habits, conduct himself in so outrageous a manner as to necessitate the use of a strait-jacket—and even then not confessing the fraud. In the investigation of these cases it is most important to determine whether the individual has any motive in simulating insanity, such as that of escaping punishment for some crime. Another point to be determined is whether the particular crime committed was incidental to a life of crime, perhaps the last act of a long series such as a hardened criminal, but not an insane person, might be expected to commit. Another point to be ascertained is whether the culprit endeavored to escape, it being well known that insane persons exhibit a perfect indifference to the consequences of their acts. It should be also remembered that insane persons never admit that they are insane; whereas, those simulating insanity are always anxious to impress every one with the fact that they are really insane.

Of the different forms of insanity, mania is that which is usually feigned by malingerers. As all maniacs are popularly supposed to be violent, the malingerer, in attempting to simulate mania, is particularly so, usually overacting the part; while the impostor, however, usually sleeps soundly, the maniac is as violent by night as by day. Dementia is less rarely simulated than mania, as it is more difficult to imitate, while the fraud is more readily recognized, being at once disclosed by the slightest reasoning power manifested by the individual.

PART III.

TOXICOLOGY.

PART III.

TOXICOLOGY.

CHAPTER I.

Frequency of Death from Poisoning—Definition of a Poison—Mode of Action of Poisons—Influence Exerted on Action of Poisons by Habit, Sleep, Disease, etc.—Evidences of Poisoning Derived from Symptoms, Post-mortem Appearances, Chemical Analysis, Experiments upon Animals, Circumstantial Evidence—Character of the Evidence the Chemical Expert may be Expected to Give in Cases of Poisoning.

In most cases of poisoning the duty of the physician making the post-mortem examination is usually limited simply to removing the stomach, intestines, etc., of the deceased person supposed to have been poisoned, and placing them in the hands of the chemist specially employed by the Commonwealth to make an examination of their contents, with the view of determining the cause of death. It is important, however, that every physician should have some knowledge of toxicology—that is, of the symptoms of poisoning, the nature of poisons, their antidotes, etc., as well as of the medical relations of the subject. The subject of toxicology, like that of insanity, is such an extensive one that its thorough consideration would demand a special treatise, far exceeding the scope of the present work. All that the author can hope to accomplish within his prescribed limits is to point out, in a very general way, what his own experience suggests as to the kind of toxicological knowledge the medical expert, who is not an analytical chemist, should possess.

The readiness with which poisons may be obtained, the facility of administering them, the close resemblance which the symptoms and post-mortem appearances of poisoning frequently bear to those due to disease, account for the fact that so many homicides and suicides are committed by this means. Indeed, statistics show that, excepting the casualties due to war, poisoning is the most frequent of all the causes of violent death. Thus, in Prussia, during the years 1869 to 1873, of 32,613 deaths, 1454 were due to poisoning.* In England and Wales, from 1863 to 1867, there were 1270 cases of poisoning.† In Massachusetts, according to the report of the State Medical Examiners, of 2976 deaths by violence, 45 were due to poisoning.‡

Definition of Poisons.—So much difference of opinion is attached to the term poison that it is difficult to define it in a way that will meet the significance attached to the word by the medical jurist as well as the layman. A poison may be defined as a substance which, introduced into the body in a state of health, by the mouth, rectum, skin, lungs, etc., ordinarily causes illness and often death, the injurious effects not being due, however, to purely mechanical action. According to the above definition, a substance would not be a poison which only affected a person when suffering from disease, like that of gastritis,

* Wharton and Stillé: *op. cit.,* vol. II, p. 5.

† "Taylor on Poisons," 1875, p. 179.

‡ "Trans. Massachusetts Medico-Legal Society," 1878–81, Cambridge.

rendering him peculiarly susceptible. Nor would fragments of glass, or iron, pins, needles, or other hard or sharp
substances be classified as poisons, even though they should
cause death when swallowed, the injurious effects experienced being due to mechanical action. It need not be
added that the particular amount, large or small, of a substance necessary to cause death affords no basis for distinguishing certain substances as poisons from others which
are not poisons. Half an ounce of oxalic acid may prove
as fatal as half a grain of strychnia.

It is not, however, a matter of much practical importance
how a poison is defined or whether the ill effect due to the
administration of some substance is regarded as poisonous
or not, since, according to law, "Whoever shall administer,
or cause to be administered, to or taken by any person,
any poison, or other destructive thing, with intent to
commit murder, shall be guilty of felony." *

Mode of Action of Poisons.—The effects of poisons
are both local and remote. In making an impression
directly upon the part of the body with which the poison
comes in contact, a poison acts locally; in affecting some
distant part of the body it acts remotely. Certain poisons
act both locally and remotely: arsenic, for example,
affecting the stomach locally and the brain remotely.
In order that a poison should produce its effects, unless
it be a corrosive, it must be absorbed—pass into the
blood.† That poisons are absorbed is proved by their
being found in the blood, brain, and viscera. The rapidity
with which this takes place will depend upon their solu-

* Taylor: *op. cit.*, p. 75.

† Christison: "Treatise on Poisons," fourth edition, Edinburgh,
1885.

bility and the relative fullness of the blood-vessels. Absorption will, therefore, be favored by bleeding or purging through depletion of the vascular system. The effects of a poison injected directly into the blood are almost instantaneous. A poison, having once passed into the blood, is carried by the latter throughout the system, being either eliminated with the bile, urine, saliva, pancreatic juice, and sweat, or deposited in the liver, spleen, kidneys, heart, lungs, brain, pancreas, muscles, or bones. Every organ would appear, therefore, to have a peculiar affinity for some one or more poisons, as shown either by the poison being excreted by a gland, as arsenic by the stomach, or by its being retained within an organ for a longer or shorter period, as lead by the brain and spinal cord.

The time required for either the elimination or the deposition of a poison varies according to the particular poison taken and to the state of the system. Potassium iodide and turpentine may appear in the urine within a few minutes after being swallowed. Arsenic may be found in the liver in four hours and earlier after it is taken, being usually eliminated from the system within fifteen days if the individual should survive for that length of time. Antimony, on the other hand, may be found four months after having been taken; lead and copper, over eight months.*

It is obvious that if a substance that is poisonous in one animal should be eliminated as rapidly as absorbed in another, but little of the toxic effect would be produced in the latter. Thus, goats are not susceptible to

* Orfila: "Annales de Hygiène publique et de Médecine legale," second series, tome III, Paris, p. 213.

the poisonous effects of belladonna, horses to that of prussic acid, on account of the rapidity with which these substances are eliminated from the systems of such animals. It is well known that, on etherizing a human being, unless more ether is inhaled than exhaled, loss of consciousness cannot be induced.

The phenomena of nutrition would lead us to suppose that it is probably only that portion of the poison flowing in the capillaries to which its effects are due. As this bears but a small proportion to that found in the stomach, which is often in large quantity, it follows that death cannot be attributed to the latter, which must be regarded as a surplus, a source of supply, should the poison circulating through the system be insufficient to produce its characteristic effects.

The exact manner in which death is caused by poison must be admitted to be as yet not understood, though the question has given rise to much discussion. The view has been advanced that poisons act in so altering the composition of the blood as to render it unfit to maintain life. Even if this could be proved, it would not be an explanation of the *modus operandi* of poisoning. In the present state of toxicological knowledge, all that can be said is that opium, for example, causes narcotism by acting upon the brain; prussic acid, asthenia through its effect upon the heart; strychnia, tetanus by its effect upon the spinal cord. As to why these particular substances act in this peculiar way, no satisfactory answer can be given, any more than as to why certain poisons are eliminated with particular secretions, as mercury with the saliva.

As a general rule, the larger the dose of the poison,

the quicker the action, the exceptions being afforded by substances like arsenic, which, when taken in an overdose, induce vomiting, and are therefore rejected from the system. Certain poisons undoubtedly act antagonistically toward each other, the effect of the one poison being more or less neutralized by the other. Thus, for example, morphia antagonizes atropia, and atropia neutralizes strychnia. Indeed, so true is this in the case of the two latter alkaloids that in strychnia-poisoning atropia should be administered as an antidote. On the same principle, digitalis might be tried in cases of aconite-poisoning, there being an antagonism between these drugs also.

Influence of Habit on Poisons.—The power of poisons to produce their characteristic effects is very much diminished by their prolonged use, enormous amounts of laudanum and morphia, for instance, being tolerated by opium-eaters, and arsenic by arsenic-eaters. Thus, it is well known that confirmed opium-eaters are able to take in one dose an amount of laudanum or morphia that would have killed them had they taken the drug in the same amount in the first instance. In the case of children drugged with opium, a common practice in the factories in England, and which is begun soon after birth, twenty drops of laudanum may be given finally at once to a child which under ordinary circumstances would be killed by a dose of five drops.

In regard to the immunity enjoyed by arsenic-eaters, it has been stated on the highest authority that peasants in Styria have been seen to swallow at once from four to six grains of arsenic without any injurious consequences being observed. Indeed, Knapp informed Maclagan that he saw a peasant swallow in his presence seven and a half grains of arsenic without ill effects.*

Influence of Idiosyncrasy.—Owing to personal peculiarities not as yet well understood, some persons are very susceptible to the action of poisons; others, again, but little so. Again, certain articles of food, such as clams, mushrooms, pork, ordinarily wholesome, will always poison certain persons if eaten, and others at times only, their systems being then temporarily disordered. The medical examiner should be on his guard, therefore, lest he attribute illness and death to the wilful administration of poison which is really due to food that was unfit to eat, or, if wholesome, acted as a poison through the peculiar susceptibility of the system at that time.

Influence of Disease.—Persons suffering with apoplexy and inflammation of the brain are very susceptible, for example, to the action of opium. On the other hand, large quantities of opium are tolerated in *mania a potu* and tetanus, Dupuytren giving, in a case of the latter disease, at one dose as much as two ounces of opium without ill effects.† It has been stated that a woman aged 29 years, affected with hemiplegia, took for six days three grains of strychnine daily without injurious consequences, the dose having been raised gradually, though one grain will usually kill a healthy adult.‡

Sleep, whether induced naturally or by opium, usually diminishes or retards the action of poisons, especially of the irritant kind.

It is well known, also, that certain animal substances,

---

* Taylor: *op. cit.*, p. 77.
† Flandin: "Traité des Poisons," vol. I, p. **231.**
‡ Taylor: *op. cit.*, p. 79.

which, when introduced into the system, are very poisonous, often indeed fatal, are, however, when swallowed, so modified by the digestive fluids as to be rendered innocuous, as shown by the fact that persons are unaffected after sucking wounds made by poisoned arrows, snakebites, etc.

Evidences of Poisoning.—The evidences in cases of alleged poisoning are afforded by the symptoms, the post-mortem appearances, chemical analysis, experiments upon animals, circumstantial evidence.

Evidence of Poisoning Derived from Symptoms.—In considering the symptoms presented by a person supposed to have been poisoned, it is most important to ascertain whether, at the time of the attack, the person was perfectly well, whether the symptoms appeared shortly after the taking of food or drink, and whether any other persons were affected in a similar manner. The great difficulty experienced by the medical examiner in determining, from the symptoms alone, whether a person has been poisoned, arises from the similarity between the symptoms of disease and those due to poison. Thus, for example, the symptoms of malignant cholera, cholera morbus, peritonitis, ulcer of the stomach, resemble very closely those due to irritant poisons. Indeed, cases of arsenic-poisoning have been mistaken for attacks of cholera morbus. On the other hand, the effects of narcotic poisons resemble in many respects those due to apoplexy, inflammation of the brain, certain cardiac disorders, etc. The above examples among many which might be given serve to prove that the symptoms alone in any case would not warrant the medical examiner in stating positively that a person had been poisoned, nor, on the other hand, in warranting him to attribute to disease an alleged case of poisoning.

Evidences from Post-mortem Appearances.—In addition to what has already been said as to the manner of making post-mortem examinations, it is especially important, in connection with poison cases, that the stomach and other viscera should be placed in a perfectly clean glass jar. Otherwise the defense on trial might plausibly argue that the poison found by the chemist was derived from the dirt in the jar, and not from the viscera of the person alleged to have been poisoned. Further, in case the stomach or other viscera are to be submitted to a chemist for analysis of their contents, the physician who makes the post-mortem examination should pack the jar with its contents securely in a box, seal the latter, and label it. It is desirable, where possible, for the medical examiner to place the box in the hands of the chemist himself. Whoever delivers it, however, should take a receipt for it. The neglect of such precautions on the part of the physician making the autopsy in a poison case may give rise, at the trial, to the objection that the stomach, etc., in passing through different hands, may have been tampered with, and the testimony of the chemist who found the poison may be thereby materially weakened. In opening the stomach in poison cases it will be found most convenient to make the incision along the lesser curvature; then, after collecting and measuring the contents, to spread the stomach out upon a clean glass plate, the inner or mucous surface being uppermost; the latter should then be examined most carefully for both lesions and the remains of the poison.

Among the post-mortem signs usually presented in

poison cases may be mentioned redness, softening of the mucous membrane of the stomach and intestines, and perforation. It is well known, however, that redness of the stomach may be due to active digestion, gastritis, use of stimulants, etc., and in some cases to a peculiar condition of the system not as yet well understood, and which might be readily attributed to the action of an irritant poison. Difference of opinion still prevails among toxicologists as to the time that may elapse before the redness of the stomach, due to an irritant poison, ceases to be recognizable and distinguishable from putrefactive changes. In this connection it may be mentioned that in a case of arsenical poisoning the reddened condition of the mucous membrane was "plainly perceptible on removing a layer of arsenic, nineteen months after interment."* Softening of the stomach cannot be regarded as characteristic in cases of poisoning, since it is only found occasionally, and is often due to natural causes, as in the case of infants. Further, in certain cases of sulphuric and carbolic-acid poisoning, the coats of the stomach were actually hardened. It need hardly be added that while perforation of the stomach, etc., as the result of corrosion or ulceration, may be due to the action of a poison, the same condition is not infrequently caused by disease.

Not infrequently remains of poison, such as crystals of arsenic, pieces of phosphorus, vegetable leaves, etc., may be found in the stomach and intestines. In cases of poisoning by prussic acid, opium, nicotine, etc., the odor of these substances, on opening the body, becomes very perceptible. Occasionally the cheeks, mouth, tongue,

* Taylor: *op. cit.*, p. 92.

and dress of the deceased may be stained, as in cases of
poisoning by mineral acids. One of the most convincing
of the evidences of poisoning that can be adduced is
the discovery of the poison.* In order to prove that
death was caused by poisoning, the law, however, does
not require that the poison should be actually discovered,
many criminals having been convicted on other evidence,
circumstantial and otherwise. Indeed, if the discovery
of the poison were essential to conviction, many criminals
would escape, as there is no reliable, certain test for many
poisons, especially of the animal and vegetable kinds.
On the other hand, the mere finding of a poison within
the stomach would not necessarily lead to conviction
if the lesions usually produced by the poison were not
present, and if other proof, such as symptoms, circumstantial evidence, etc., were absent. Indeed, it might be
argued, in such a case, that the poison had been introduced
into the stomach after death for some malicious purpose,
with the motive, perhaps, of exciting suspicion and of
leading to the conviction of some innocent person. The
fact that the poison was found in the liver, spleen, etc.,
would be a much stronger proof that death was caused
by the poison than the finding of it in the stomach alone,
as in the former case it would be inferred that the poison
had been absorbed. It must be remembered, however,
that a poison might be introduced into the stomach or
rectum after death, and thence by osmosis pass possibly
all through the body, for, although the bony cranium
and spinal column would prevent osmosis, nevertheless,
if the poison were imbibed by the nerves, it might possibly

---

* "Tunc demum res certa, erit, ubi venemum ipsum reperietur
facile agnoscendum" (Wharton and Stillé: *op. cit.*, vol. ii, p. 44).

be transmitted by the latter not only to the cord, but even to the brain itself.

Evidence from Chemical Analysis.—In making an analysis it is important that the chemist should inform himself as to the nature of the symptoms, as well as of the post-mortem appearances presented, inasmuch as these may serve, to some extent at least, to indicate the nature of the poison taken. In every case the analysis should be made as carefully and as thoroughly as possible. As a matter of precaution only one portion of the suspected substance should be analyzed at a time, the remaining portion being reserved in case an accident should happen, or there should arise a necessity for future investigation. The substance suspected to be poison ought to respond to all the tests. It is also important that the reagents, previous to being used, should have been determined to be pure, so-called "chemically pure" reagents often containing impurities. In many analyses it is of advantage to reduce the bulk of the liquid by evaporation, since the quantity of poison present might be so small as not to respond to the ordinary tests. Notwithstanding, how-ever carefully the analysis may have been made, the chemist fails in many instances to discover any poison. It must be remembered, in connection with failures to find poison in those cases where all the other evidence concurs in showing that poison had been taken, that the latter may have been vomited or have passed out of the system in the feces and urine. The poison, further, may have been of such a nature as to be unrecognizable by any means at present known, or to have been decom-posed in the blood or tissues during life or after death.

Evidence from Experiments on Animals.—In those cases

where the poison cannot be determined by either the symptoms, post-mortem appearances, or chemical analysis, there remains still another resource—that of experimentation upon animals. For example, in an obscure case of strychnia-poisoning, some of the suspected matter, found perhaps in the stomach of the deceased, should be injected subcutaneously into a frog, the latter animal, as is well known, being extremely susceptible to the effects of that alkaloid.* Criminals have been convicted of giving strychnia, aconitia, etc., in this way, such poisons having been recognized through their characteristic effects produced upon animals. It is an interesting fact, in this connection, that animals enjoy an immunity from being poisoned by certain plants which, when eaten by man, usually prove fatal; and, further, that man may be poisoned by eating an animal that has previously fed upon such plants. Thus, it is well known that the milk of cattle browsing upon the herbage in certain parts of South America, and the meat of the rabbit which has eaten belladonna, will prove poisonous to human beings partaking of them.†

Circumstantial Evidence.—Although the consideration of the circumstantial evidences of poisoning in a criminal case does not constitute a part of the duty of the medical examiner, nevertheless a knowledge of all the circumstances bearing upon the case will be of advantage. Among such circumstances may be mentioned particularly: Whether the person accused had any motive for poisoning the deceased. Was there any evidence

* Orfila: "Traité des Poisons," troisième edition, tome premier, Paris, 1826, p. 31.
† Guy and Ferrier: *op. cit.*, p. 372; Beck: *op. cit.*, vol. ii, p. 414.

that the accused had recently purchased the particular poison found, or that he had had any in his possession for some time? Did he give the deceased always his meals? Was medical advice sought, and, if so, was the medicine always given by the accused? If any matters were vomited during the illness of the deceased, were they submitted to the physician, for examination, or thrown away at once and nothing whatever said about them? Was the burial premature and very quiet? Was an autopsy objected to? It is needless to say that, if the accused acted in such a way, there would be good reason, indeed, to suspect foul play.

Character of Evidence of the Chemical Expert.—In all criminal cases of poisoning the physician or the chemist, or whoever makes the analysis, must be prepared to answer at the trial such questions as the following: Could the sickness or death be ascribed to poison, and, if so, to what particular poison? Would such a poison as that alleged to have been given produce death if administered in sufficient quantity? At what period was the poison given? Could such a poison disappear so entirely from the system as to leave no trace? Might the poison discovered in the body of the deceased have been derived from some other source than that which was claimed to show that it had been criminally administered? * The answers to be given by the medical witness to such questions will largely depend upon what particular kind of poison may have been given, as will become more apparent when the different kinds of poisons will have been considered.

* Tardieu, A.: "Etude médico-legale et clinique sur l'Empoison-nement," Paris, 1867.

The effects of poison are simulated occasionally; the imposture will be discovered, however, in time at least, if not by other means. Insane people are frequently deluded with the idea that attempts are being made to poison them, or that they have been poisoned.

CHAPTER II.

Classification of Poisons—Irritant Poisons—Poisoning by Mineral
Acids, by Alkalies and their Salts, Noxious Gases—Poisoning by
Phosphorus, Arsenic, Antimony, Mercury, Lead, Copper, etc.—
Poisoning by Oxalic Acid, Carbolic Acid, etc.—Poisoning by
Decomposed Food, Ptomaïnes, Neurotic Poisons—Poisoning by
Opium, Alcohol, Ether, Chloroform, Chloral, Nux Vomica,
Strychnia, Belladonna, Stramonium, Tobacco, Lobelia, Hydro-
cyanic Acid.

SYSTEMATIC writers upon the subject of toxicology vary
very much in the manner in which they classify poisons.
In this manual, however, poisons will be regarded as consisting of only two kinds: IRRITANTS and NEUROTICS.*

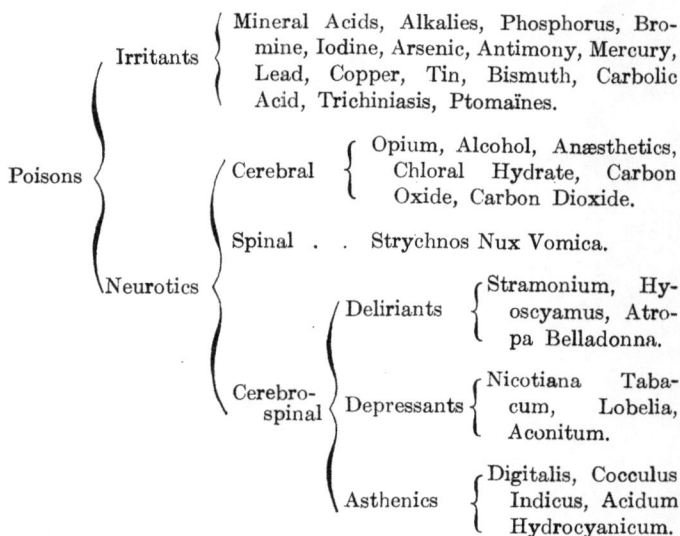

Poisons
- Irritants: Mineral Acids, Alkalies, Phosphorus, Bro-
mine, Iodine, Arsenic, Antimony, Mercury,
Lead, Copper, Tin, Bismuth, Carbolic
Acid, Trichiniasis, Ptomaïnes.
- Neurotics
  - Cerebral: Opium, Alcohol, Anæsthetics,
Chloral Hydrate, Carbon
Oxide, Carbon Dioxide.
  - Spinal . . Strychnos Nux Vomica.
  - Cerebro-spinal
    - Deliriants: Stramonium, Hy-
oscyamus, Atro-
pa Belladonna.
    - Depressants: Nicotiana Taba-
cum, Lobelia,
Aconitum.
    - Asthenics: Digitalis, Cocculus
Indicus, Acidum
Hydrocyanicum.

* Taylor: *op. cit.*, p. 78.

Irritant poisons include substances which, when swallowed, give rise to an acrid, burning taste, followed by nausea, vomiting, cramps in stomach, purging, the matters vomited and purged being often mixed with blood, these symptoms being due to inflammation of the mucous membrane of the alimentary canal, terminating not infrequently in ulcer, perforation, and gangrene. They may possess simple irritant properties or specific ones, and are derived from the mineral, vegetable, and animal kingdoms. The simple irritant poisons include such substances as the mineral acids and alkalies. Among those possessing specific properties may be mentioned phosphorus, arsenic, antimony, mercury, oxalic and carbolic acids, cantharides, poisoned meat, fish, etc.

Neurotic poisons include such substances as have a specific action upon the brain and spinal cord, causing headache, giddiness, drowsiness, stupor, delirium, coma, convulsions, paralysis. They are derived from the vegetable kingdom and include substances like opium, chloral, strychnia, atropia, Calabar bean, prussic acid, etc.

IRRITANT POISONS.

Poisoning by Mineral Acids.—As a general rule, most cases of poisoning due to mineral acids are accidental in character, suicide being only occasionally committed by such means, and homicides but rarely. As the symptoms, post-mortem appearances, general treatment, in poisoning by the different mineral acids, are very much the same, they may be conveniently considered together. The symptoms in cases of poisoning of this kind, which depend more on the degree of concentration than on mere quantity, are a burning sensation in the mouth, followed by violent

17

pain in the stomach, vomiting of dark-colored coffee-grounds-like matters containing blood, and occasionally portions of mucous membrane.

In those cases in which *concentrated sulphuric acid,* or oil of vitriol, comes in contact with the larynx or the mucous membrane of the air-passages, œdema of the glottis may set in immediately, death soon following.

In all cases of poisoning by mineral acids, magnesia, chalk, plaster off the walls (if nothing better), soap-suds, oil, milk, mucilaginous drinks, flaxseed tea, or barley-water may be administered. If undiluted acid has been swallowed, however, there is but little hope that the remedies just mentioned or any others will do much good, though a case has been reported in which sulphuric acid given by injection, by mistake for castor oil, was followed by recovery. The smallest recorded quantity of sulphuric acid known to have destroyed life was one drachm, the shortest known period at which death has taken place being within two hours.* On the other hand, cases have occurred in which stricture of the esophagus caused by sulphuric acid was delayed till two years after the taking of the poison.

On post-mortem examination stains and corrosions are found on all parts with which the acid has come in contact. The skin is stained black or dark brown. The stomach is filled with black, yellow, or brown fluid, perhaps distended with gas, its mucous membrane charred or inflamed, perforation not being uncommon in cases of sulphuric-acid poisoning. In cases of sulphuric-acid poisoning the contents of the stomach should be filtered and then treated with any soluble salt of barium. The

* Christison: *op. cit.,* p. 162.

dense white precipitate produced, insoluble in acid and alkalies, with charcoal and blowpipe will yield barium sulphide, which in turn with a mineral acid gives sulphuretted hydrogen, recognizable by the black stain it gives to filtering paper dipped into a solution of lead salt.

As the symptoms produced by swallowing *nitric acid* or aqua fortis do not differ essentially from those caused by sulphuric acid, it will not be necessary to dwell upon them further than to say that the skin is stained yellow by nitric acid, not black or brown, as by sulphuric acid.

In cases of poisoning by nitric acid, the matters obtained from the stomach should be first filtered. The clear acid liquid so obtained should then be heated and a weak solution of potassium carbonate added. Paper dipped into a concentrated solution of the latter will afterward burn with deflagration. A few drops of the filtered solution evaporated to dryness on a glass slide will give crystals of potassium nitrate. On making a solution of these crystals and adding a crystal of ferrous sulphate with a drop or two of strong sulphuric acid, the green color of the crystal will change to reddish-brown, due to the formation of ferric sulphate. Morphia and brucia will serve as tests for concentrated nitric acid, being turned red by the acid. Ruddy brown fumes are also given off when nitric acid is poured on copper.

The smallest quantity of nitric acid recorded as having destroyed life is 2 drachms, as in the case of a boy aged 13 years, who died in thirty-six hours. Death usually takes place, however, within twenty-four hours, though a case has been reported in which poisoning from nitric acid proved fatal in one hour and three-quarters. Although most cases of nitric-acid poisoning are due to accident, nevertheless murder has been committed in this way. Thus, a man was convicted in 1889 of pouring a mixture of nitric and sulphuric acids down the throat of a woman whilst in bed, nitro-cellulose produced by the action of the above mixture upon cotton and wood being found by the medical examiner upon the clothes of the deceased and the wood of the floor on which the murder was committed.*

The symptoms of poisoning by *hydrochloric acid*, commonly known as muriatic acid, spirit of salt, are essentially the same as those caused by nitric acid. The parts, however, with which the acid first comes in contact, more especially the skin and fauces, are colored white, not yellow.

In order to extract hydrochloric acid from the stomach, it is only necessary to add silver nitrate to the filtered contents, the white precipitate of silver chloride formed being readily recognizable by being soluble in liquor ammoniæ and precipitable by nitric acid, blackening upon exposure to light and melting into a mass known as horn silver when heated. The fact that hydrochloric acid dissolves gold leaf in the presence of nitric acid affords a convenient test for the concentrated acid, as also the white fumes given off with vapor of ammonia.

The smallest quantity of hydrochloric acid known to have destroyed life is half an ounce,† death taking place in eighteen hours, the average period being about twenty-four hours. Cases of hydrochloric-acid poisoning have, however, been reported in which life was prolonged for even two months after the taking of the poison. As a

* Taylor: *op. cit.*, p. 104.
† Taylor: *op. cit.*, p. 104.

rare occurrence, murder is committed by means of hydrochloric acid, as in a well-known case when the acid was poured down a child's throat by her stepmother, who so confessed after her condemnation.*

Poisoning by Alkalies.—As potassa and soda are so extensively used in the arts, in the manufacture of glass and soap, under the name of pot- and pearl-ashes, soda ashes and soap lees, eau de Javelle (chlorinated soda colored red with peroxide of manganese), and ammonia in the form of aqua ammoniæ for various household purposes, death has frequently occurred as the result of taking them accidentally, and in some cases, though more rarely, suicidally.

The symptoms of poisoning by the alkalies are an acrid, nauseating taste, followed by a burning heat in the throat and stomach, violent abdominal pains, vomiting, and purging. Ammonia, being more irritating than potassa or soda, affects the respiratory organs especially, inducing a choking sensation. In cases of poisoning by any of the alkalies, vinegar and water, lime or orange juice, oil, which forms with alkali soap, should be given, opium being administered to relieve pain. The quantity of potassa or soda or ammonia that may prove fatal is variable, death having been caused by half an ounce of caustic potassa and by 40 grains in solution and by 2 drachms of ammonia. Persons have, however, recovered after swallowing over an ounce of ammonia. Death may take place from poisoning by alkalies within a few hours or days. It has been stated that ammonia in the form of vapor has caused death even in as short a time as four minutes,† and that a boy died in

* Orfila: "Ann. d'Hygiene," tome xi, p. 35.
† Woodman and Tidy: *op. cit.*, pp. 92, 105.

three hours after swallowing three ounces of a strong solution of carbonate of potassium.* On the other hand, in some cases of alkali-poisoning life may be prolonged for several months. In fatal cases, on post-mortem examination, the mucous membrane of the mouth, throat, and gullet will be found corroded, often blackened, and even completely destroyed, the larynx and bronchi being particularly inflamed and softened in cases of ammonia-poisoning.

In examining the contents of the stomach, as a general rule, the organic matters can be removed by evaporation and subsequent heating; the ash remaining being digested with distilled water and filtered, the potassa or soda will be found in solution as a carbonate. Potassium compounds give a violet color; sodium compounds, a yellow color to the smokeless flame of spirit or gas. The presence of these alkalies can be readily recognized also by means of the spectroscope. Potassium can also be tested for by using tetrachloride of platinum, which throws down a yellow granular precipitate consisting of potassio-platino-chloride. In making use of this test, the absence of ammonia must be insured. Soda may be recognized from the white precipitate thrown down by the addition of potassium antimoniate. Ammonia may be extracted from the stomach by distilling about one-fourth of the liquid, the vapor being carried through a bent tube into a well-cooled receiver containing a small quantity of water acidulated with hydrochloric acid. If no ammonia should be given off, the contents of the retort should be treated with alcohol filtered and redistilled with calcium hydrate, by which free ammonia, perceptible from its odor, will be obtained. As

* Taylor: *op. cit.*, p. 111.

ammonia is one of the products of putrefaction, if the contents of the stomach should be found in that condition it will be useless to attempt to make an analysis. A convenient test for ammonia is platinum tetrachloride, which gives a yellow precipitate.

The alkaline salts and earths, potassium nitrate or saltpeter, used in medicine and in the manufacture of gunpowder, potassium bitartrate or cream of tartar, potassium sulphate, chlorinated soda and potash or bleaching salts, magnesium sulphate or Epsom salts, the salts of barium, strontium, calcium, and alum, have all proved fatal when taken in overdoses or in large quantities. As cases of poisoning from such substances were not homicidal in character, but resulted from accident,* it will not be necessary to describe the symptoms, post-mortem appearances, etc. It may be mentioned, however, that the proper treatment in such cases, generally speaking, is to evacuate the poison by emetics and mucilaginous drinks, and the administration of antiphlogistic remedies.

Poisoning by Noxious Gases.—Among the irritant poisons may also be included nitrous acid, sulphurous acid, hydrochloric acid, and chlorine gases. The deleterious effects of the fumes of such gases are well known, causing irritation and inflammation of the throat, eyes, and air-passages, inducing in some cases even spasm of the glottis. The production of these gases is incidental to various manufacturing processes, nitrous acid gas being generated upon a large scale in water-gilding and brass button-making, sulphurous acid gas in bakers' ovens, hydrochloric acid gas in potteries. As such cases of poi-

* Taylor: *op. cit.*, pp. 113, 115 ; Wharton and Stillé: *op. cit.*, vol. II, pp. 110, 112, 114, 122.

soning are often of a chronic rather than acute character, and but rarely become the subject of medico-legal investigation, it will not be necessary to dwell further upon them.

Poisoning by Phosphorus.—With the description of phosphorus-poisoning we begin the consideration of that class of irritant poisons which not only act upon the mucous membrane of the alimentary canal, or the part of the body they come directly in contact with, but also upon remote parts of the system, the nervous centers being often especially affected. It is true that some of the alkaline and earthy salts just mentioned possess similar properties to some extent; but, as poisoning is rarely caused in this way, their specific properties were not referred to. Phosphorus is but seldom used for homicidal and not very frequently for suicidal purposes. It may be mentioned in this connection that cases have been reported in which attempts have been made to murder individuals, or even whole families, by putting phosphorus, in the form of a vermin-killer, etc., in the tea or soup, their lives being saved, however, by the smell or luminosity caused by the poisonous substance.

Most cases of poisoning of this kind are accidental in character, caused by swallowing the phosphorus paste used for destroying vermin, or the tops of lucifer matches. Poisoning by phosphorus is much less common than formerly, the red or amorphous form, which is not poisonous, being so much more used than the yellow variety. In acute cases the symptoms vary at the commencement, sometimes setting in rapidly, at others being protracted. As a general rule, within from one to two hours a peculiar, disagreeable taste is experienced, accompanied with intense warmth in the stomach and bowels, which gradually turns into a violent, burning pain. Eructations having a garlicky odor, followed by nausea, vomiting, and purging, are not infrequent. The matters vomited are usually dark-colored, and have the garlicky odor of phosphorus. The pupils are dilated, the abdomen distended, the extremities cold, the pulse weak, the thirst intense. Between the third and fifth days, if the case is a protracted one, jaundice appears, often accompanied by retention of urine and by delirium, the patient dying possibly in convulsions or comatose. Recovery is very rare. The most constant symptoms in chronic phosphorus-poisoning are weakness and fatigue, pains in the abdomen, with diarrhœa, intermittent toothache, carious teeth, with gums swollen and distended with pus; the complexion sallow, eruption upon the skin; falling off of the hair, increase of phosphates in the urine.

There is no chemical antidote for phosphorus. The poison should be removed as soon as possible. If the patient is seen shortly after taking the poison, the stomach-pump should be used; otherwise, an emetic of sulphate of zinc or sulphate of copper should be administered, the latter being given in three-grain doses, well diluted, at intervals. Magnesia or chalk, in gruel, should be given. If the poison has had time to reach the intestines, purging should be tried; on no account should oil be given, as the phosphorus would be dissolved, and its absorption greatly promoted. It has been stated, nevertheless, that oil of turpentine may be advantageously used as an antidote in cases of phosphorus-poisoning.*

It is most important, as a precautionary measure, that

* " Bull. Gén. de Thérapeutique," tome LXXVIII, p. 169.

those engaged in phosphorus manufactories should be extremely cleanly in their habits, changing their clothes after work, washing their faces and hands, and rinsing their mouths with some slightly alkaline wash. Saucers filled with turpentine should be placed about the factory, the fumes appearing to exert a protective effect. The smallest quantity of phosphorus known to have destroyed life was one and a half grains in a man, one-eighth of a grain in a woman. The one-fiftieth of a grain has, however, killed a child. Death in cases of acute phosphorus-poisoning usually takes place within a period of from three to six days. In one case recorded death occurred in half an hour. On the other hand, cases have been reported where one child swallowed a teaspoonful of phosphorus paste and another sucked three hundred matches and yet both recovered.* In chronic cases of phosphorus-poisoning life may be prolonged for months or even for years.

On post-mortem examination the mucous membrane of the alimentary canal is usually found inflamed, softened, and discolored. In chronic cases the most important change observed is the fatty condition of the liver, kidneys, heart, muscles, etc., the fat being probably derived from the albumin of the tissues. The best way of extracting phosphorus from the stomach is that of Mitscherlich. This method consists in distilling the suspected fluid in the dark with a small quantity of dilute sulphuric acid, the object of the latter being to neutralize the ammonia developed during putrefaction. The vapors are made to pass through a tube kept cool by running water into a receiver, a flash of light appearing every time that the phosphorous vapor condenses in the tube. This method is so

* Woodman and Tidy, *op. cit.*, p. 71.

delicate that one part of phosphorus may be detected by it in one hundred thousand of substance.

Bromine and iodine, like phosphorus, are irritant poisons, possessing specific properties as well. The only case of fatal bromine-poisoning known to the author is that of a daguerreotypist who committed suicide at Williamsburg, New York, by swallowing an ounce by weight of this substance.* Murder has been attempted by putting iodine in the food, but was unsuccessful owing to the discoloration caused by the poison exciting so much suspicion that it was not eaten.

The symptoms of poisoning by bromine are spasmodic action of the muscles of the larynx and pharynx, with great difficulty in breathing, followed by burning pain in the stomach. An ounce of bromine has caused death in seven hours and a half. Iodine in large doses causes a burning heat in the throat, pain in the abdomen, vomiting, purging. In such cases emetics should be administered. The post-mortem appearances presented are those of an irritant poison. Fatal results have followed from the taking of twenty grains of iodine.† Death occurs usually within thirty hours after the taking of the poison. It may be mentioned that caution should be exercised by the physician in prescribing iodide of potassium, as some persons are very susceptible to its influence. In such cases, headache, abdominal pain, thirst, inflammation of the nostrils and eyes, salivation, pustular eruption, follow its administration even when given in small doses.

Poisoning by Arsenic.—Arsenic is found in nature in the metallic form, or in combination with other metals,

---

* "New York Med. Journal," 1850.
† Woodman and Tidy: *op. cit.,* p. 86.

such as zinc, copper, iron, and with sulphur in the form of orpiment and realgar. Arsenic is extensively used in the arts, in the manufacture of enamel, glass, composition candles, vermin-killers, fly-powders; ship-builders protect their timber from worms, farmers preserve their grain, grooms improve the coats of horses, and women their skin, by arsenic.* Arsenic is so readily obtained and so easily administered, and is so easily suspended in tea, coffee, milk, and soup, etc., that it is of all poisons the most frequently used for homicidal and suicidal purposes. Of the various preparations of arsenic, the important ones, medico-legally, are the white oxide commonly known as arsenious acid, the yellow sulphide or orpiment, the green arsenite of copper or Scheele's green, the liquor potassæ arsenitis or Fowler's solution. In whatever form taken, though, whether solid, liquid, or gaseous, or howsoever applied, either as a wash, an ointment, or a plaster, arsenic acts as a poison.

While a case has been reported in which murder was committed by means of metallic arsenic,† arsenious oxide, or white arsenic, is the form of arsenic most commonly made use of for poisoning purposes. Arsenious oxide occurs in commerce as a heavy, white, opaque, or translucent powder, or in masses. It is nearly tasteless, and but slightly soluble in cold water, only one-half of a grain being dissolved by an ounce of water; the solubility is increased by hot water, alkali, but diminished by organic matter. As a general rule, the symptoms of arsenical poisoning develop gradually, being usually delayed for from half an hour to an hour, or even longer. In certain

* Guy and Ferrier: *op. cit.*, p. 436 ; Tardieu: *op. cit.*, p. 323.
† Casper: "Vierteljahrs.," October, 1854.

cases, especially when a large dose has been taken, poisonous symptoms may appear almost immediately. The countenance expresses depression and great suffering. A burning pain is experienced in the pit of the stomach, which is increased by pressure; vomiting is invariably present, the matters vomited consisting of a white gumlike substance or of a brown liquid mixed with bile or blood. Diarrhœa is usually present, accompanied with pains at the anus; severe cramps are felt in the legs. The throat is hot and constricted, the tongue furred, and thirst is intense. The skin is hot and dry, the head aches, the pulse is rapid and small. The conjunctivæ are reddened, the eyes smart and are suffused, and light is dreaded. Though there are usually extreme restlessness and nervous twitchings, the mind, as a general rule, is clear. Death may occur with convulsions of an epileptiform character, or may resemble, as already mentioned, that of cholera morbus. In some cases death takes place very quickly, as if due to shock. The symptoms in chronic cases of arsenic-poisoning, as, for example, where workmen have been exposed to the vapors of arsenic, are much less pronounced than in acute ones. The eyes are inflamed and watery; headache, giddiness, vomiting, diarrhœa, may be present; the skin is affected with an eczema; there may be some local paralysis; salivation and even mania have been noticed.

In cases of arsenical poisoning, if the patient is seen soon after taking the poison, the stomach-pump should be used. If any length of time has elapsed, however, hot milk and water emetics of sulphate of zinc and mustard should be given. If there has been much vomiting, eggs and milk and magnesia, with sugar in milk, should be administered, the latter forming an insoluble compound with arsenious oxide. Stimulants should be given in a state of collapse, and anodynes for nervousness. The antidote in most repute in cases of arsenical poisoning is the hydrated sesquioxide of iron, by which the arsenic is converted into the insoluble arseniate of iron. It can be freshly and quickly prepared by diluting the tincture of the chloride of iron, adding ammonia in excess, collecting the precipitate on filtering paper, and carefully washing and administering at once when moist. The hydrated sesquioxide of iron so prepared should be given in large doses and frequently, followed later by a dose of castor oil. Freshly precipitated hydrated peroxide of magnesium has also been proved serviceable as an antidote. Nitrate of potassium may be given, also, in repeated doses in order to promote the elimination of the poison by the kidneys. It appears that, however large the amount of arsenic taken, no more than two grains need be absorbed to cause death. At all events, that amount has proved fatal, though there have been recoveries after much larger doses. Death usually takes place within twenty-four hours, though it may occur within twenty minutes or be delayed ten to sixteen days after taking the poison.*

On post-mortem examination the mucous membrane of the stomach will usually be found highly inflamed, presenting, in some cases, a uniform deep red color; in others, only red patches. In some cases the mucous membrane is thickened; in others, softened and easily separated, but not usually either ulcerated or gangrenous. Perforation rarely, if ever, occurs.† While arsenic appears to have

---

* Taylor: *op. cit.*, p. 130.

† Orfila: "Médecine Légale," tome III, p. 330.

some specific effect upon the stomach, not infrequently the small intestine, the cæcum, and the rectum are inflamed as well. It must be mentioned that in some cases of arsenic-poisoning there is an entire absence of any signs of inflammation, even though there had been symptoms of inflammation during life.

Arsenic is not a cumulative poison, being only temporarily deposited in the liver and other organs, and rapidly eliminated in the urine and other secretions; accordingly, no trace of it is likely to be found after death, should the person have survived two or three weeks after taking the poison. On the other hand, arsenic, as is well known, being a powerful antiseptic, at least in many cases, the bodies of persons poisoned by this means may be so well preserved, as already mentioned, as to admit of the detection of the poison months and even years after burial. Under such circumstances the absence of cadaveric odor is noticeable, and there will be frequently observed numerous yellow patches on the abdominal viscera, due to the formation of yellow sulphide of arsenic through the action of sulphuretted hydrogen upon arsenious oxide. In examining the contents of the stomach, the examiner should first carefully look for solid particles of arsenious oxide in the walls of the stomach itself, as well as among its contents. The stomach should then be cut into small pieces with a perfectly clean pair of scissors, and, together with its contents, placed in a clean porcelain evaporating dish. Distilled water, with one-sixth its bulk of pure hydrochloric acid, should be added, and the whole gently boiled for about an hour, by which time most of the solid portions of the mixture will be disintegrated. After cooling, the mixture should be filtered, the filtrate being afterward concentrated over a water-bath. In order to extract arsenic from the liver, spleen, or other organs, the tissues should be very finely cut up, and, after being treated with distilled water and hydrochloric acid, must then be filtered.

The different tests for arsenious oxide may be regarded as being of three kinds—solid, liquid, and what may be called special tests. Of the solid tests the three following will be found convenient and easy of application: The first test consists in heating upon charcoal the suspected substance; if the latter be arsenious oxide, the odor of garlic will become very perceptible. The second test is to slowly heat the substance in a narrow glass tube until it sublimes; if arsenious oxide be present, there will be formed on the cool part of the tube a white ring of octahedral crystals (Fig. 47), which can be seen by a good magnifier.

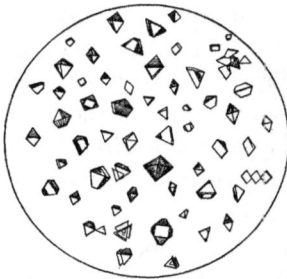

Fig. 47.—Crystals of arsenious oxide by sublimation, magnified 30 diameters.

It is true that calomel and corrosive sublimate will produce white rings under the same circumstances, but they will not consist of octahedral crystals. The third test is to heat the suspected substance in a reduction-tube (Fig. 48), about three inches long and an eighth of an inch in diameter, with dry sodium carbonate and charcoal, the flux being in the proportion of about four to one of the substance examined and intimately mixed with it. If arsenious oxide be present, it will be reduced, metallic arsenic being condensed as a brilliant steel-gray ring upon the lower part of the tube. That the ring so formed does consist of arsenic is still further shown by the fact that it is entirely soluble in sodium hypochlorite.

The liquid tests are the ammonio-sulphate of copper, the ammonio-nitrate of silver, and sulphuretted hydrogen. Ammonio-sulphate of copper, when added to a solution of arsenious oxide, throws down a light green arsenite of copper, the precipitate being soluble in ammonia and free acids. The characteristic color does not appear immediately if the arsenic is in very small quantities. The ammonio-sulphate of copper, when used for this purpose, should be freshly prepared by adding to a somewhat dilute solution of sulphate of copper just enough liquor ammoniæ to throw down a pale blue precipitate. Ammonio-nitrate of silver gives to a solution of arsenious oxide a canary yellow precipitate of arsenite of silver soluble in an excess of ammonia. The reagent can be freshly prepared by adding just enough liquor ammoniæ to a solution of nitrate of silver to precipitate the brown oxide of silver. It should be

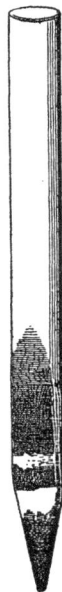

Fig. 48.—Ordinary reduction-tube, with two sublimates; the upper, brownish black; the lower, the pure metal in an annular deposit.

mentioned, however, that as various organic matters which might be present in the contents of the stomach will produce similar colors with both copper and silver, the precipitates of arsenite of copper and silver obtained by the liquid tests should be submitted to further tests,

18

such as that by the reduction method just described.
The sulphuretted hydrogen test consists in passing washed
sulphuretted hydrogen gas through the solution of the
suspected substance slightly acidified with hydrochloric
acid.　If arsenious oxide be present, there will be precipitated the yellow tersulphide of arsenic, soluble in alkalies,
but insoluble in acids.　In dilute solutions the excess of
gas may have to be driven off before the precipitate is
separated.　The sulphide of arsenic so obtained should still
further be tested by subliming it with a reducing agent.
It should be mentioned, in connection with this test, that
somewhat similar precipitates are yielded by cadmium, tin,
and selenium in the presence of sulphuretted hydrogen.
For all practical purposes the cadmium sulphide need only
be considered in this respect, and it should not even prove
a source of fallacy; it is distinguished from arsenic sulphide
in being soluble in acids and insoluble in alkalies, and
further in forming a brown oxide instead of a ring when
dried and oxidized on charcoal.

The special tests for the detection of arsenious oxide are
known as Marsh's and Reinsch's tests.　The principle of
Marsh's test is based upon the fact that arsenious oxide is
decomposed in the presence of nascent hydrogen, arseniuretted hydrogen gas being formed from which the arsenic
can be obtained as a brilliant steel or brown-gray deposit
in the form of rings.　The simplest method of performing
Marsh's test is first to generate perfectly pure hydrogen
gas and then to add to the materials generating the latter
the solution suspected to contain arsenious oxide.　The
hydrogen gas may be generated by putting strips of chemically pure zinc and diluted sulphuric acid into a suitable
glass vessel provided with two mouths.　Through one of

the mouths a glass tube should pass down vertically below the surface of the liquid, and through the other mouth a tube bent at right angles by means of which the hydrogen gas generated may issue. The gas should be dried by allowing it to pass through a tube containing pieces of fused calcium chloride or pumice-stone moistened with sulphuric acid, then through a horizontal tube of hard German glass about a foot long, turned up at the farthest end and terminating in a small point, so that the gas as it escapes will burn in a jet. It is most essential, before lighting the jet of gas, that all atmospheric air be excluded from the tubes, otherwise a violent explosion will ensue. After waiting a sufficient length of time the gas may be lighted, and it will burn with a faintly luminous, scarcely perceptible flame. The purity of the materials used in generating the hydrogen gas must now be demonstrated. This is accomplished

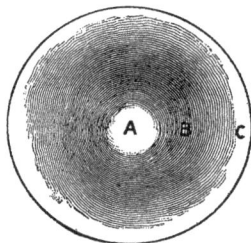

Fig. 49.—Deposit obtained by Marsh's apparatus: A, Metal; B, mixed deposit; C, arsenious oxide.

by applying the flame of a large spirit-lamp to the horizontal glass tube until it becomes red hot. Should no stain or deposit occur just beyond the heated spot, or no deposit form on a piece of white porcelain held over the burning jet, the absence of arsenic is assured (Fig. 49). A small quantity of the suspected solution being now introduced through the vertical tube, any arsenious oxide present will be decomposed, arseniuretted hydrogen will be set free, and will burn with a pale blue flame, white fumes being frequently evolved having an alliaceous odor. If the latter be made to pass into a short, wide glass tube, they will condense as a white powder, sometimes crystalline in form, recognizable as arsenious oxide. If a white porcelain plate be now placed over the flame of the arseniuretted hydrogen, a deposit is formed consisting of three concentric rings, the inner ring being metallic arsenic, the middle ring arsenic and arsenious oxide, the outer ring arsenious oxide.

It should be mentioned, in connection with Marsh's test, that antimony in the presence of hydrogen will yield a deposit very similar to that due to arsenic. The arsenical deposit can, however, be distinguished from the antimonial one, as the former is soluble in a solution of chlorinated lime, but insoluble in hydrochloric acid, whereas the latter is insoluble in chlorinated lime, but soluble in hydrochloric acid. Further, if the deposit of arsenious oxide be converted into arsenic acid by the addition of nitric acid, and the latter be treated with ammonio-nitrate of silver, the brick-red arsenite of silver will be formed, affording another proof of the presence of arsenic. On placing the flame of a large spirit-lamp just below the horizontal tube, which should have been contracted after heating it in several places, when it becomes nearly red hot a deposit of metallic arsenic will be formed just in advance of the flame, the deposit continuing to increase until it may occupy the whole of the contracted space, or even part of the tube in advance of the latter. This deposit constitutes what is known as the *arsenical mirror*, and should be exhibited in court as proof that arsenic had been found.

Reinsch's test consists in boiling bright strips of copper in a hot solution of the suspected substance previously acidulated by hydrochloric acid. Metallic arsenic being deposited upon the strips of copper, the latter are then withdrawn and placed in a reduction-tube and the presence of arsenic demonstrated in the manner already described. The freedom from arsenic of the copper strips used in Reinsch's test is shown by the fact that they are not tarnished after having been boiled in hydrochloric acid.

It must be admitted, however, that the value of Reinsch's test, in cases of arsenical poisoning, has been exaggerated, since antimony has also been obtained in the form of octahedral crystals by this process. Thus, in a well-known case of a woman accused of murder by poisoning with arsenic, the octahedral crystals presented in court by the defense were stated by the chemist retained by the prosecution to be arsenic, whereas as a matter of fact the octahedral crystals in question had been obtained from antimony. The woman was, of course, acquitted at once.*

Nevertheless, Reinsch's process for the determination of the presence of arsenic is still useful as a preliminary test, the presence of organic matter not interfering with it. Further, the crystals of antimony obtained by this means are not always octahedral, but often prismatic, the deposit violet, the sublimate amorphous and insoluble in water, whereas the sublimate of arsenic is steel-gray and slightly soluble in water.

Aceto-arsenite of copper, or Brunswick green, also known as Vienna emerald or Paris green, not infrequently causes death by poisoning, this pigment being extensively used in the staining of wall-paper, toys, bonbon papers, in coloring artificial flowers, articles of dress, bonnets, etc. Cases of arsenical poisoning from this pigment are usually chronic in character, resulting from living in rooms whose walls are covered with this green paper, the fine dust from which, getting into the lungs, produces the poisonous ef-

* "Medico-Legal Journal," vol. xiv, No. 1, p. 81.

fects. Death may also result from overdoses of Fowler's solution or liquor potassæ arsenitis, from arsenic acid, Scheele's green or arsenite of copper, and orpiment, or the yellow sulphide of arsenic.

In all cases of alleged arsenical poisoning the medical examiner should thoroughly satisfy himself that the arsenic obtained could not by any chance have been conveyed into the body of the deceased in the solid or liquid food. The importance of such caution being exercised is shown by the fact that certain kinds of beer, especially in England, have been stated in recent years to contain beer arsenic, and in quantity greater than would have been supposed.

Poisoning by Antimony.—Of the different preparations of antimony, the potassio-tartrate, or tartar emetic, is the most important medico-legally, though the chloride has not infrequently been also a cause of death. The symptoms of antimonial poisoning are a strong metallic taste during the act of swallowing, heat, soreness, and constriction of the throat, pain in the stomach, followed by nausea, vomiting, and diarrhœa. The pulse is quick and small, the skin is cold and clammy, cramps are often present in the extremities. The urine is often increased in quantity, but voided with pain. Death may take place during the stage of prostration, which is very intense, or may be preceded by delirium and convulsions. Insensibility is sometimes produced by the taking of large doses.

The symptoms of tartar-emetic poisoning resemble in many respects those of cerebro-spinal meningitis; indeed, so much so that in a celebrated case a woman who was accused of committing murder by means of tartar emetic was acquitted, to a great extent at least, on the ground that the prosecution had failed to prove that death was due to tartar emetic and not to cerebro-spinal meningitis.

Cases of chronic poisoning by antimony are characterized by great weakness and exhaustion, accompanied by nausea, vomiting, and purging. In cases of antimonial poisoning, should vomiting not have been induced by the poison, the fauces should be tickled and hot water and milk administered, the stomach-pump being used as a last resource. As soon as the poison has been removed from the stomach, strong coffee should be given, followed by opium.

The antidotes are any substances that contain tannin, such as cinchona bark, green tea, infusion of nutgalls, and decoction of oak bark, etc. As well known, infants and young children tolerate large doses of tartar emetic, especially when suffering from diseases of the larynx and lungs. Three-quarters of a grain has, nevertheless, proved fatal in a child,* and two grains in an adult.† The recoveries reported after the taking of large doses were without doubt due to the poison having been rejected by the stomach, vomiting having been promptly induced. Death may take place within a period varying from seven hours to a few days, though it may not take place for many months. The post-mortem appearances usually found are inflammation of the mucous membrane of the stomach and intestines, and in some cases of the brain and lungs. The liver is frequently enlarged and softened, and appears to undergo a fatty degeneration.

It is well known that antimony causes a fatty degeneration of the liver in animals. The peasants in Brunswick, Europe, avail themselves of a knowledge of this fact, and

---

* Guy and Ferrier: *op. cit.*, p. 473.
† "Archives Gén.," tome xxvi, p. 262.

feed their geese upon white oxide of antimony, to make them fat and well flavored. It should be mentioned, however, in connection with the structural changes caused by antimonial-poisoning, that cases have been reported in which post-mortem examination failed to reveal a lesion of any kind.*

Tartar emetic, when heated by the spirit-lamp, decrepitates and chars; and if the blowpipe is used, the metal is reduced. If a drop of the solution of tartar emetic be evaporated on a glass slide, a crystalline deposit will be left which, when examined by a lens or a microscope, will be found to consist of tetrahedral crystals or of some derivative of the octahedron (Fig. 50).

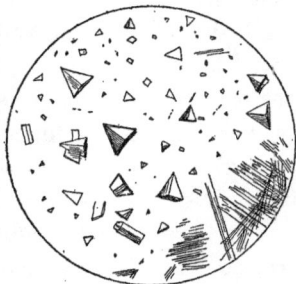

Fig. 50.—Crystals of tartar emetic; × 30.

In the extraction of tartar emetic from the stomach the contents of the latter should be diluted with water, filtered, and acidulated with tartaric acid, and then sulphuretted hydrogen gas passed through the liquid, by which means the orange tersulphide of antimony, which is soluble in sulphide of ammonium, will be precipitated. Should antimony fail to be detected by this method, then Marsh's or Reinsch's test should be tried, antimoniuretted hydrogen being generated if the first process be used, instead of arseniuretted hydrogen as in the case of the test being used for the detection of arsenic. Antimony is absorbed in the system, and may be found in the viscera, blood, urine, the

* "Archives Gén.," September, 1865; "Boston Med. and Surg. Journal," 1865.

same methods being made use of as in the case of arsenical poisoning. If the quantity of antimony suspected to be present is very small, a coil of pure zinc-foil wound around a platinum foil may be suspended in a weak acidified solution, when the metallic antimony will be deposited upon the platinum. The deposit so obtained should now be washed and digested in nitric acid until it is dissolved, and the solution evaporated. The residue, being acidified, should then be treated with sulphuretted hydrogen. It may be mentioned, in this connection, as tartar emetic is very often prescribed medicinally, in the form of wine of antimony, compound syrup of squill, proprietary and patent cough medicines, that the medical examiner should be very cautious in attributing death to poison in case of finding this salt in the stomach, unless it were obtained in quantity far exceeding that of ordinary doses.

The symptoms and post-mortem appearances presented in cases of poisoning by terchloride or butter of antimony resemble rather those produced by mineral acids than by tartar emetic. Terchloride of antimony when thrown into water yields a copious white flaky precipitate, the oxychloride or powder of Algaroth. The latter is soluble in tartaric acid, and turns orange-red when touched by sulphide of ammonium.

Cases have been reported in which butter of antimony has been used for suicidal and homicidal purposes. Thus, in one instance an army surgeon swallowed intentionally between two and three ounces of this poison and died in ten hours and a half. In 1883 a woman and her daughter were tried at the Worcester Assizes, England, for killing the illegitimate child of the latter with terchloride of antimony, but were acquitted on the ground that the prosecution had failed to prove administration of the poison.*

Poisoning by Mercury.—While all the mercurial compounds, corrosive sublimate, calomel, red and white precipitates, red oxide, etc., are more or less poisonous, bichloride of mercury, or corrosive sublimate, from a medico-legal point of view, is the most important.

The symptoms in cases of acute mercurial poisoning usually appear immediately after the poison is taken, a burning pain being at once felt, extending from the throat to the stomach. The face becomes flushed. The mouth and tongue look white and shriveled, as if they had been thoroughly painted with silver nitrate. The breathing is difficult, the pulse thready. The abdomen is painful and swollen, the pain being increased upon pressure. The stools are bloody. The thirst is intense, and a white, stringy, or bloody mucus is vomited. The urine is more or less suppressed. The skin is cold and clammy. Salivation usually sets in about the third day. Death generally takes place soon after collapse, though it may be preceded by convulsions and coma.

The symptoms of poisoning by corrosive sublimate resemble more closely those of arsenic than any other poison; the local action of the former, however, as its name implies, is corrosive in character; that of the latter, irritant.

The antidotes, white of egg, or wheat flour mixed with milk, should be given at once, and in most cases continued two or three times daily for some weeks. The white of one egg may be considered as sufficient to neutralize four grains of corrosive sublimate. As the vapors of mercury are poisonous when inhaled, it not infrequently happens

* Taylor: *op. cit.*, p. 163.

that those who are engaged in working mercurial ores, in looking-glass plating, water-gilders, barometer-makers, are poisoned in this way, the fumes being given off from the metal even at ordinary temperatures. Such cases are usually chronic in character. The symptoms begin with nausea and vomiting. Coppery taste in the mouth and pains in the stomach are constantly occurring. The breath becomes fetid and swallowing difficult. A hacking cough sometimes follows, with hæmoptysis. Ultimately salivation becomes very noticeable. The margins of the gums sometimes present a blue line like that observed in lead-poisoning, the gums being red, painful, swollen, and even ulcerated. Tremors and convulsive movements of the limbs finally become well marked, and the patient soon dies unless actively treated. The smallest quantity of corrosive sublimate known to have proved fatal is three grains.* Death usually takes place within a period varying from three to six days, though it has occurred within half an hour in some cases, and been protracted in others more than two weeks.

On post-mortem examination the salivary glands are found enlarged. The abdomen is usually tympanitic. The mucous membrane of the mouth and throat presents a grayish-white color, at times being exceedingly inflamed or corroded, or even in a sloughy condition. The stomach is often very much inflamed, and is frequently covered with a slate-colored layer of finely divided mercury, or, in cases of putrefaction, with a black precipitate of sulphide of mercury. The intestines and urinary bladder are often also much inflamed. In order to determine the presence of mercury in the stomach, the contents of the latter should

* Taylor: *op. cit.*, p. 146.

be mixed and crushed in a mortar, alcohol being added to facilitate filtration. The mixture, being acidified with hydrochloric acid and gently warmed, should then be filtered, and the filtrate tested by sulphuretted hydrogen and Reinsch's test. In order, however, to obtain corrosive sublimate from the stomach, the contents should be concentrated by evaporation, and then shaken with a large bulk of ether, which is a powerful solvent of corrosive sublimate. The ether must then be carefully decanted and distilled at a gentle heat, the residue being then appropriately tested. Corrosive sublimate may be found in the urine within two hours and in the saliva within four hours after taking the poison. In examining the urine about fourteen ounces should be evaporated down to one ounce and acidified and filtered. The filtrate should then be boiled with a piece of bright copper and placed in a reduction-tube. The saliva may be tested by observing whether a piece of bright copper becomes tarnished when placed in saliva acidulated with hydrochloric acid. Among the tests for the mercurous salts may be mentioned liquor calcis, which throws down a black precipitate (black wash). Iodide of potassium gives an olive-green precipitate; chromate of potassium gives a bright red precipitate. With mercuric salts liquor calcis gives a yellow precipitate (yellow wash). With corrosive sublimate liquor ammoniæ gives a white precipitate. Iodide of potassium gives the scarlet iodide of mercury.

From a medico-legal point of view it is important for the practitioner to bear in mind that the symptoms of mercuric salivation closely resemble those due to cancrum oris, or gangrene of the mouth, as suits for damages have been brought against physicians by their patients on the charge that they had been poisoned by the mercury administered, when they were really suffering from one or other of the diseases just mentioned.* Indeed, suits for malpractice have been instituted in which it was afterward shown that no mercury in any form whatsoever had been prescribed. In cases of this kind the chemical analysis of the saliva would at once settle the question.

Cases have also been reported in which death was caused by nitrate of mercury. In one instance this poison was put in a pudding with homicidal intent, and in another case suicide was committed by its means.

Poisoning by Lead.—The most important salts of lead, from a medico-legal point of view, are the acetate and carbonate, though other preparations of lead are used for medicinal purposes. Cases of acute lead-poisoning are very rare, and when they occur result from accident. Soon after swallowing acetate of lead, or sugar of lead, a metallic taste, dryness in the throat, and thirst are experienced. The most prominent symptom, however, is severe colicky pain, which is intermittent, but is relieved by pressure. Constipation is invariably present, the muscular coat of the intestines being paralyzed. The urine is scanty and red; cold sweats, cramps, paralysis of the lower extremities, appear as the case progresses, followed often by tetanic spasms and convulsions.

In treating cases of acute lead-poisoning emetics should be given, and if vomiting should not be induced by these means, then the stomach-pump should be resorted to. The antidotes are the soluble alkaline and earthy sulphates; the sulphate of magnesium is the best, and should be administered with eggs, opium being given to allay pain.

* Christison: *op. cit.*, p. 412.

The amount of acetate of lead that would prove fatal, and the length of time that would elapse before death took place, are uncertain. Cases of chronic or slow lead-poisoning or saturnine poisoning are of very frequent occurrence, owing to the various ways in which lead in one form or another may be introduced into the system. It may be swallowed in drinking-water or applied in the form of cosmetics or hair-dyes, or inhaled in the form of fumes, as by artists, painters, plumbers, and workmen engaged in the manufacture of white lead.*

The symptoms that appear first in chronic cases are collectively known as lead colic, among which the blue line at the margin of the gums is very characteristic, and those later as lead palsy. On post-mortem examination in cases of acute lead-poisoning, inflammation of the alimentary canal may be found; but, not infrequently, no lesion of any kind is present. In cases of chronic poisoning no special lesion is found, with the exception that the intestines are usually in a contracted condition and the muscles specially affected flabby. Lead, however, is found in the bones, brain and spinal cord, and viscera. In extracting lead from the stomach the contents should be treated with dilute nitric acid in order to form nitrate of lead, the latter being then treated with sulphuretted hydrogen. If the lead has, however, been rendered insoluble by any organic matters normally present, or by the antidotes, the contents of the stomach should be first incinerated, and the ash treated in the manner just mentioned. The black precipitate so obtained can be shown to contain lead by reducing it by means of charcoal and the blowpipe.

Poisoning by Copper.—The salts of copper are rarely

* Guy and Ferrier: *op. cit.*, p. 494.

used for homicidal or suicidal purposes. Most cases of poisoning by copper result from accident, being caused, for example, by keeping food or cooking in copper vessels. Green carbonate of copper, or natural verdigris, is formed under such circumstances, and is very poisonous. All the salts of copper are poisonous. The sulphate, or blue vitriol, and the subacetate, or artificial verdigris, are the most important from a medico-legal point of view. In large doses sulphate of copper is a powerful emetic; fatal results are often on that account prevented, the poisonous matters swallowed being at once rejected by the stomach. Among the other symptoms presented are thirst, abdominal pain, purging, suppression of urine, jaundice. In cases of copper-poisoning, vomiting, should be induced, or the stomach-pump resorted to in case the poison has not produced that effect. White of egg, mixed with sugar and milk, should be freely administered. On post-mortem examination the body will be found to present a yellow color. The mucous membrane of the stomach is usually inflamed, and its contents are of a blue color. An ounce of sulphate of copper has proved fatal; but the quantity necessary to destroy life, as well as the period at which death occurs, is variable.* In extracting a salt of copper the contents of the stomach should be evacuated and treated with dilute hydrochloric acid and filtered, the filtrate being then treated with sulphuretted hydrogen. The blackish-brown precipitate of sulphide of copper should then be converted into the nitrate by the addition of nitric acid, and the latter salt tested. A convenient test for salts of copper is liquor ammoniæ, which gives a blue precipitate; the latter, when dissolved in an excess of ammonia, forms a beautiful sapphire-blue.

* Woodman and Tidy: *op. cit.*, p. 175.

Poisoning by Zinc, Bismuth, etc.—Cases of poisoning from zinc are comparatively rare. Of the different preparations, the sulphate and chloride, the latter often used as a disinfectant, need only be considered. The symptoms of poisoning by zinc resemble those due to sulphate of copper. Half an ounce to an ounce has proved fatal. In some instances death has occurred within fourteen hours. The post-mortem appearance presented is inflammation of the alimentary canal. The best antidote is albumin. Bismuth, more particularly the subnitrate, deserves mention on account of its being frequently adulterated with arsenic. Indeed, the finding of arsenic, when the cause of death was alleged to be poisoning, has been accounted for on the supposition that it was given in the subnitrate of bismuth administered.* With respect to the preparations of chromium, it should be mentioned that not infrequently fatal cases of poisoning have resulted from persons eating cakes and buns colored yellow by means of chromate of lead. Although the various preparations of tin, iron, silver, gold, and manganese may all prove fatal when taken in large doses, as they are so unlikely to be used for poisoning purposes, and of thus becoming the subject of medico-legal inquiry, their special consideration can be dispensed with.

Poisoning by Oxalic Acid.—Of the irritant poisons of vegetable origin, oxalic acid is the most important. Resembling sulphate of magnesium or Epsom salts, for which it is readily mistaken, and being easily procured either as oxalic acid or as salt of sorrel, salt of lemons, potassium oxalate, it is not infrequently taken by accident or for suicidal purposes. The symptoms of poisoning by

* Wharton and Stillé: *op. cit.*, vol. II, pp. 269, 283.

oxalic acid are a hot, burning, acid taste during swallowing, followed by pallor, clammy perspiration, extreme
prostration, abdominal pain, accompanied with vomiting.
If the poison be diluted, the vomiting may be protracted.
In some cases, however, there is no vomiting at all; in
others it may continue incessantly until death. The nervous system appears to be also remotely affected, as, in
cases of recovery from oxalic-acid poisoning, spasmodic
twitchings of the facial muscles, temporary loss of voice,
numbness and tingling of the legs, have been observed.   In
treating cases of oxalic-acid poisoning, magnesia, plaster
from the walls, chalk or carbonate of calcium, should be
given; the last is the best remedy, as it forms with oxalic
acid the inert calcium oxalate. Vomiting should afterward be induced by an emetic of sulphate of zinc.   Alkalies and their carbonates should not be given, however,
under any circumstances, as the salts formed would be as
poisonous as the oxalic acid. The mucous membrane of
the mouth, tongue, and throat appears as if bleached. The
stomach is often black, and even gangrenous, though perforation is rare. It often contains a dark brown liquid.
Sixty grains of oxalic acid have proved fatal.*   Death may
take place very quickly,—within ten minutes,—or may be
protracted several days.

A convenient test for oxalic acid is calcium sulphate,
which gives a white precipitate of calcium oxalate soluble
in mineral, but insoluble in vegetable acids.   In cases when
the amount of oxalic acid is so small that it will not redden
litmus paper, its presence can be detected by adding nitrate
of silver, a white precipitate of oxalate of silver being
formed which is completely dissolved by nitric acid.   The

* Taylor: *op. cit.*, p. 108.

presence of oxalic acid in an organic liquid can be readily demonstrated by means of dialysis. Thus, if a solution of calcium sulphate be placed within the tube of the osmometer (Fig. 51) and the fluid supposed to contain the oxalic acid in the outside jar, the oxalic acid will osmose through the membrane on the end of the tube and will form inside the latter crystals of oxalate of calcium, readily recognizable under the microscope by their octahedral form (Fig. 52). The method most frequently made use of, however, in obtaining oxalic acid from either the contents

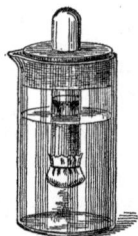

Fig. 51.—Osmometer.

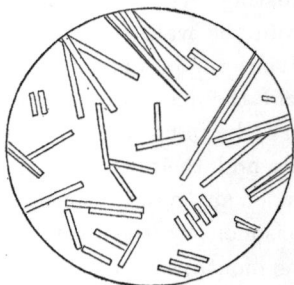

Fig. 52.—Crystals of oxalic acid;
× 30.

of the stomach or the matters vomited, is by the addition of acetate of lead to the contents of the stomach previously filtered. Oxalate of lead is precipitated; the latter being treated with sulphuretted hydrogen, oxalic acid is set free, and the lead is precipitated as sulphide of lead.

It may be mentioned, in this connection, that both tartaric and acetic acids have proved fatal when taken in doses of an ounce. In the treatment of such cases, magnesia, chalk, or the alkaline carbonates may be given.

Poisoning by Carbolic Acid, Phenic Acid, Phenol.—Carbolic acid, sometimes called coal-tar creasote, is so extensively used as an antiseptic and is so powerful a poison that it demands at least brief mention. The symptoms of poisoning are vertigo and intoxication, accompanied by intense burning pain in the mouth and stomach, with vomiting of frothy mucus. The pupils are contracted; the pulse rapid and intermittent. The urine is frequently suppressed; whatever is passed is dark-colored and smoky; convulsions and coma often supervene. In treating such cases oil and demulcent drinks, sulphate of sodium or Glauber's salts may be administered, and the stomach-pump should be used. With any treatment, however, there is but little chance of recovery. Six or seven drops having caused the most dangerous symptoms, it is to be expected that death will follow almost immediately after the taking of any large quantity. Indeed, death has been known to take place within three minutes after swallowing about an ounce of carbolic acid,* though life may be protracted two or three days.† As a general rule, after death the mouth, esophagus, and stomach are found white and corroded. The lungs are usually found much congested; the brain occasionally so. Carbolic acid can be usually found in the urine by agitating the latter with an excess of ether, removing the ether by means of a pipette and evaporating. The minute oily residue left has the character of that acid. The best general test for carbolic acid is probably its odor.

Poisoning by Vegetable Substances.—There are a number of well-known substances, such as croton oil, the oil of the seed of Croton tiglium (Fig. 53), ergot of rye, the fool's parsley (*Æthusa cynapium*), elaterium obtained from the wild cucumber, water dropwort (*Œnanthe crocata*),

* "Phila. Med. Times," vol. ii, p. 284.
† Woodman and Tidy: *op. cit.*, p. 515.

castor-oil beans, seeds and wine of colchicum (Fig. 54), cowbane (*Cicuta virosa*), oil of savin procured from the tops of Juniperus sabina, yellow jessamine, veratrum viride, and the other species of Colchicaceæ, all of which possess poisonous properties of an irritant character. As cases of poisoning by these substances are usually accidental in character and unlikely to become the subject of medico-

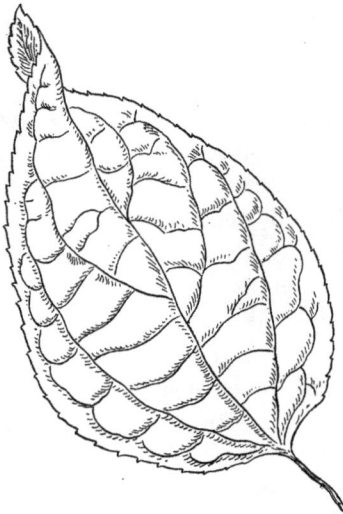

Fig. 53.—Leaf of the Croton tiglium.

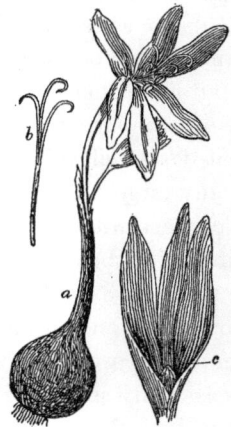

Fig. 54.—Colchicum autumnale: *a*, Flowering plant; *b*, stigmas; *c*, leaves and fruit.

legal inquiry, except in the case of oil of savin, often used as an abortive, it will not be necessary to dwell upon their characteristic properties.

Poisoning by Eating Fungi.—The symptoms caused by eating poisonous fungi, often resembling those due to poison administered with homicidal intent, demand some consideration on the part of the medical jurist. As is well known, while certain fungi may be eaten usually with impunity, there are others which invariably prove poisonous. The symptoms which follow the eating of poisonous mushrooms, and which usually appear within an hour, are giddiness, thirst, abdominal pain, vomiting, purging, sweats, dimness of vision, delirium, convulsions, and coma.* Death usually takes place within twenty-four hours. In treating such cases the stomach-pump should be used and an emetic of sulphate of zinc and castor oil should be administered. On post-mortem examination the stomach and intestines are usually found inflamed and may even be gangrenous. The contents of the stomach should be carefully searched for the gills and spores of the mushroom suspected to have been the cause of poisoning, the particular fungus being by these means identified.

Poisoning by Decomposed Food.—The irritant poisons of animal origin are cantharides and the poisons developed under certain circumstances in food. The symptoms of poisoning from the powdered *Cantharis vesicatoria* (Fig. 55), or the tincture of cantharides, are pain in swallowing, a burning sensation in the mouth and stomach, thirst, vomiting, and bloody stools, priapism, inflammation and swelling of the genitalia, and occasionally convulsions and delirium. In treating a case of poisoning from such a cause, emetics and thick warm liquids should be administered, opiates should be given in the form of enema, and suppositories and leeches applied. On post-mortem examination the mucous membrane of the alimentary canal and urino-genitary tract will be found inflamed. Portions of the wings and wing-cases of the insect, which resist putrefac-

* Casper: *op. cit.*, vol. ii, p. 61.

tion for a long time, should be looked for, especially in the large intestine. An ounce of the tincture of cantharides has proved fatal, death taking place in twenty-four hours.

Poisoning by Micro-organisms, Bacteria, etc.—Apart from trichinosis produced by eating raw pork, the muscular tissue of which is infested with the minute worm, the *Trichina spiralis* (Fig. 56), poisonous effects are frequently produced by eating food in a state of putrefaction

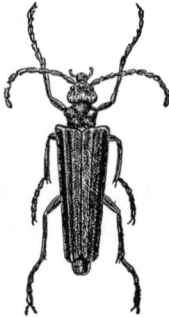

Fig. 55.—Cantharis vesicatoria (Spanish fly).

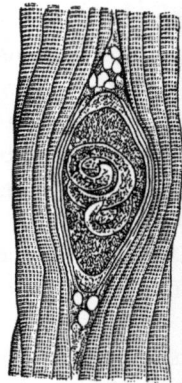

Fig. 56.—Trichina spiralis, coiled within its cyst ($\times$ 50).

induced by micro-organisms, bacteria, etc., or food containing *ptomaïnes* or "cadaveric alkaloids," so called on account of the manner of their production and of their effects when introduced into the system.* The poisonous effects frequently produced by eating meat, sausage, cheese, fish, mussels, have been proved to be due to the presence of either micro-organisms or ptomaïnes.† The

---

* V. C. Vaughan and F. G. Novy: "Cellular Toxins," Philadelphia, 1902, p. 29.

† Vaughan and Novy: *op. cit.*, pp. 189, 193, 213.

symptoms and post-mortem appearances in all such cases are those of an irritant poison,—giddiness, nausea, cramps, vomiting, purging,—the mucous membrane of the alimentary canal being found inflamed. As to what particular micro-organism the changes developed in food should be attributed to, making it poisonous; as to the exact nature of the ptoma͞nes which cause poisoning when introduced into the system in some persons, but give rise to no inconvenience whatever in others, considerable difference of opinion still prevails among bacteriologists and toxicologists. It is to be regretted, particularly from a medicolegal point of view, that so little has been definitely established with reference to the nature of such organisms and poisonous principles, inasmuch as attempts might be made, in cases of undoubted poisoning, to account for the latter on the supposition that the person was poisoned by the food eaten rather than by the poison actually administered with homicidal intentions. On the other hand, innocent persons might be accused of having committed murder by means of poison when death in reality was due to poisoned food.

NEUROTIC POISONS.

With opium we begin the consideration of neurotic poisons, or that class of poisons which affect more particularly the great nervous centers—the brain and spinal cord. The symptoms produced by neurotic poisons are usually headache, giddiness, drowsiness, stupor, delirium, convulsions, paralysis, there being, however, little or no inflammation of the mucous membrane of the alimentary canal, as was seen to be so common in cases of poisoning by irritants. The post-mortem changes in cases of neurotic poisoning are but few, and not well marked—more or less fullness of the cerebral vessels being observed, but rarely accompanied with effusion of serum or blood in the brain.

Cerebral Neurotics.—*Poisoning by Opium.*—In addition to the different preparations of opium that are used medicinally there are a number of patent medicines which contain this drug or some of its alkaloids, among which may be mentioned Godfrey's cordial, Dalby's carminative, Winslow's soothing syrup, Locock's pulmonic wafers, Battley's liquor, etc. It is on this account that so many cases of poisoning are due to opium, the drug being taken, in one form or another, either accidentally or suicidally, or administered to others with homicidal intent.

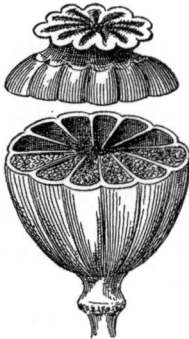

Opium, the concrete juice of the unripe capsule of the poppy (*Papaver somniferum*, Fig. 57), is a complex substance containing a number of active principles, the chief of which are morphia, meconic acid, narcotina, codeia, narceine, thebaine, papaverine.

Fig. 57.—Papaver somniferum (capsule of the opium poppy).

From a medico-legal point of view, however, morphia and meconic acid are the most important of these principles, as by their reactions the presence of opium is recognized.

The symptoms of opium-poisoning are giddiness, drowsiness, stupor, profound sleep; flushed face, slow and stertorous breathing; eyes closed and pupils contracted, insensible to light; pulse rapid and small or free and slow; skin moist and cool. The patient, from being aroused and kept awake only with difficulty, soon passes into a completely comatose condition, death taking place from apoplexy, collapse, convulsions, though usually tranquilly. These symptoms may appear within a few minutes after taking the drug, or be protracted for several hours, according to the condition of the system and the mode of administration. Opium, as is well known, is absorbed more rapidly when the stomach is empty than when full; when the person is at rest than when taking exercise; and in a liquid rather than in a solid form. The effects of taking opium habitually and for a long time are emaciation, loss of appetite, constipation, failure in mental and physical vigor, neuralgic pains, premature old age, and death. The smallest quantity of opium known to have produced death is four grains.* The amount that can be taken without producing death, however, by those persons habitually using opium is almost incredible. Indeed, Quincey is said to have taken as much as nine ounces daily. Death may take place within an hour or be delayed several hours. If the patient survives over twelve hours, the chance of recovery is good.

The post-mortem changes in cases of opium-poisoning are neither well marked nor constant. Occasionally the cerebral vessels are found in a turgid condition, with some subarachnoid effusion of serum at the base of the brain or around the spinal cord.

In treating cases of poisoning by this substance, the opium should be removed by means of the stomach-pump as soon as possible, or by an emetic, such as sulphate of zinc or mustard water. Cold water should be dashed over the face and chest in order to overcome the increasing lethargy. Strong coffee should also be administered, and

* Christison: *op. cit.*, p. 713.

the patient, to be kept aroused, must be made to walk between two attendants. Atropia should be administered hypodermically, the effects upon the pupils being carefully watched. Should all such remedies fail, then electro-magnetism may be resorted to. The symptoms of poisoning by morphia, the most important of the principles of opium, differ only from those produced by the drug itself in manifesting themselves sooner and in tending to produce convulsions more frequently. One grain of morphia has in more than one instance proved fatal, and less than a grain when administered hypodermically.* The external application of morphia has also been followed by fatal results when applied to an abraded surface. The post-mortem appearances presented in cases of morphia-poisoning do not differ from those already described as being caused by opium.

There is no direct chemical test for opium. As every watery solution contains, however, meconate of morphia, if the latter salt can by any means be shown to exist in the contents of the stomach, the vomit, or the tissues, then in this indirect way the presence of opium may be considered as having been demonstrated. The principle of the analysis is based upon the possibility of decomposing the meconate of morphia that may be present, and then re-obtaining the acid and salt constituting the alkaloid † as meconate of lead and acetate of morphia. The process consists in filtering the contents of the stomach—any solid matters being finely divided and well mixed with liquid. If acetic acid

* Wharton and Stillé: *op. cit.,* vol. ii, p. 338.

† For a detailed account of the methods made use of by Staas and Dragendorff for the detection of alkaloids in suspected matters, see Wharton and Stillé, *op. cit.,* vol. ii, p. 354.

be added and then acetate of lead, meconate of lead will be precipitated, acetate of morphia remaining in solution. The mixture is then filtered and tested in the following manner: The solution containing the acetate of morphia is divided into two parts. To one part is added a solution of perchloride of iron, by which a greenish-blue color is produced. To the other part, evaporated to dryness, nitric acid is added, by which a yellow color becoming orange-red is developed. The precipitate containing the meconate of lead is diffused in water, through which sulphuretted hydrogen is then passed, by which sulphide of lead is precipitated and meconic acid left in solution. To the latter, on the addition of perchloride of iron, a blood-red solution will be formed. It must be remembered, however, that even in cases where there was every reason to suppose that opium had been given, and when the analysis was made with the greatest care, not a trace of either meconic acid or morphia could be found.

Poisoning by Cocaine.—Cocaine, the alkaloid of the leaves of the erythroxylon coca, so much used by physicians in late years as an analgesic, may cause even in doses of one-sixth of a grain, toxic symptoms when injected hypodermically. Indeed, it has been stated that in some instances death has resulted from cocaine-poisoning, the symptoms being nausea, vomiting, loss of vision, cramps, convulsions, delirium. The cocaine-habit now so common has already been referred to in connection with the subject of life insurance.

Poisoning by Alcohol.—The poisonous effects of alcohol are of either an acute or a chronic character. The symptoms of acute alcoholic poisoning are unsteadiness of gait, incoherent talking, stupor, and coma. The features have a vacant expression, or may be suffused and bloated. The lips are livid, the pupils are unusually dilated, bloody froth appears upon the lips, the breathing becomes difficult and then stertorous. In treating such cases emetics should be administered, or the stomach-pump used, cold affusions employed, and ammonia and coffee given. On post-mortem examination the mucous membrane of the alimentary canal, the lungs and brain may be found congested, with serous effusion under the arachnoid and in the ventricles.

Alcoholism, or chronic poisoning by alcohol, as already mentioned, is the proximate cause of numerous diseases, such as cirrhosis of the liver, fatty liver, epilepsy, gastritis, disease of the kidneys. Alcoholism indirectly favors the production and the mortality of disease in general by diminishing the resisting power of the system. The perceptions finally become blunted, the moral and intellectual faculties are perverted by its habitual use, until at last the victim becomes a dipsomaniac. Alcohol can be obtained from the stomach by distillation. The contents of the stomach, if acid, having been neutralized by sodium carbonate, should be distilled. The distillate, having been mixed with calcium chloride, must be then redistilled. The second distillate should then be shaken up with dry sodium carbonate, the supernatant fluid being drawn off for testing purposes.

Poisoning by Anæsthetics.—The cerebral neurotics include the anæsthetics ether, chloroform, and chloral hydrate. The symptoms produced by *ether* are very much the same as those of alcohol. When inhaled, slow, prolonged, stertorous breathing results, the surface of the body feels cold, the lips become blue, the face pale. The pulse is at first accelerated, but is afterward slowed. The muscles become relaxed. The eyes are fixed and glassy, the pupils dilated. Anæsthesia becomes deep, coma following with entire loss of sensation. Nausea and vomiting frequently occur. In poisoning by liquid ether, the stomach-pump should be employed, emetics being given afterward. When inhalation has been carried too far, the patient should have plenty of fresh air, cold affusions should be applied, and artificial respiration and galvanism resorted to. Congestion of brain and lungs, and the heart-cavities filled with liquid, dark blood, are usually found upon post-mortem examination. The mode of extracting ether from the contents of the stomach is the same as that made use of in the case of alcohol.

The symptoms produced by *chloroform* when swallowed are those of an irritant poison, but when inhaled the symptoms resemble those caused by ether, but appear much more rapidly. Death is caused by paralysis of the respiration and circulation, the nerve-centers being probably directly affected, as death in some cases is almost instantaneous. In treating cases of chloroform-poisoning, if the chloroform has been taken in a liquid form, an emetic should be resorted to, or the stomach-pump used, and stimulants administered. If the chloroform has, however, been inhaled, with the first dangerous symptoms it should be instantly discontinued and fresh air admitted, as a few drops of chloroform may prove fatal in as many seconds. Water should be dashed in the face, the tongue pulled out, artificial respiration practised, and the galvanic current applied. The post-mortem appearances presented in cases of chloroform-poisoning are those of death due to asphyxia. Chloroform can be extracted from the stomach by distillation and tested by passing the vapor through a flame, by which it will be decomposed into carbon, hydrochloric acid, and chlorine. The carbon will be recognized by its black deposit, the acid by reddening litmus, and the chlorine by applying starch-paper dipped in a solution of potassium iodide; the latter being decomposed and the iodine set free, the starch will become blue.

Chloral hydrate, so much used at the present day to procure sleep, is on that account not infrequently a cause of death, overdoses being taken accidentally. In cases of poisoning by it the face becomes flushed; the pupils, at first contracted, are then dilated; the pulse is quick; profound sleep is induced, which passes rapidly into coma through cessation of the circulation and respiration. The action of chloral hydrate may be possibly due to its decomposition in the system, probably in the blood, into an alkaline formiate and chloroform. As thirty grains of chloral hydrate have proved fatal, that amount can hardly be considered a safe dose to begin with.* Nevertheless, a case has been reported in which as much as four hundred and sixty grains were supposed to have been swallowed and yet the patient recovered.†

Among the cerebral neurotics should be included carbon monoxide and carbon dioxide, as the effects of both these gases when inhaled are very similar to those produced by narcotic poisons. Carbon monoxide is produced when charcoal is burned, and frequently collects in pits, cellars, wells, and mines. Carbon dioxide, as is well known, is one of the principal products of respiration. The symptoms of poisoning by both these gases are essentially the same—

* Taylor: *op. cit.*, p. 209.
† "Philadelphia Medical Times," October 15, 1870.

giddiness, headache, drowsiness, insensibility, and coma being the most prominent.

In treating cases of carbon monoxide poisoning, venesection and transfusion of arterialized, defibrinated blood should be tried. In cases of poisoning by carbon dioxide the patient should be given plenty of fresh air, the cold douche, galvanism, and stimulants applied, artificial respiration practised, etc. It will be found much more difficult, however, to revive a person affected by carbon monoxide gas than by carbon dioxide, the poisonous effects of the latter being transitory, whereas carbon monoxide, in displacing the oxygen carried by the red corpuscles of the blood and forming a somewhat stable compound with the hæmoglobin of the latter, renders resuscitation difficult.

Suicides are frequently committed, more especially in France, by inhaling charcoal vapor; and death is often caused accidentally in America in the same way, as in those cases where persons have gone to sleep in a room with a charcoal fire burning without a flue. The absorbing effect of carbon monoxide blood upon light transmitted through it has already been referred to in connection with the spectroscopic examination of blood.

Spinal Neurotics.—*Poisoning by Strychnia.*—Strychnia, one of the most important of poisons on account of being so frequently taken accidentally or suicidally, as well as given with homicidal intent, exists, together with brucia, in the seeds of the strychnos nux vomica, a tree found in India. The seeds owe their poisonous properties to these two alkaloids, and as the symptoms of poisoning, etc., by nux vomica are the same as by strychnia, we may pass at once to the consideration of the latter—merely mentioning that thirty grains of nux vomica (about the

Toxicology.

weight of one seed) and three grains of the alcoholic extract have proved fatal.* Strychnia is not only used
medicinally, but is readily obtainable otherwise, entering
largely into the composition of the so-called "vermin-
killers," Battley's vermin-killer containing as much as 23
per cent.

The first symptoms of strychnia-poisoning, appearing
usually within from ten to twenty minutes after it is taken,
the poison being so rapidly absorbed, are a general uneasi-
ness and restlessness, followed by a feeling of suffocation.
The muscles begin to twitch and the head and limbs to
jerk, and then violent tetanic convulsions come on, involving the whole body. The legs are stretched out stiffly
and separated, the feet arched and turned in, the arms are
flexed and drawn across the chest. The head and body
are so bent back that opisthotonos supervenes, the patient
resting upon his head and heels. The respiratory movements are arrested by the muscular spasm, the face becomes livid, the pupils dilated. The muscles of the mouth
are so contracted as to give rise to a broad grin, the risus
sardonicus, and lockjaw is frequently present, though one
of the later symptoms. Intense thirst may be experienced.
The paroxysm may last from half a minute to several
minutes; subsiding, it is followed by relaxation, the patient being bathed in perspiration and utterly prostrated.
In a short time, sometimes within a few minutes, the
paroxysm returns, being brought on by the slightest cause
—a breath of wind, a slight noise, an effort to move. It
increases in frequency and violence; death results usually
in between five and six hours from asphyxia or exhaustion,
the mind remaining clear almost to the last. As small a

* Christison: *op. cit.*, p. 201.

quantity as the one-sixteenth of a grain of strychnia has proved fatal in a child, and one-half of a grain in an adult.* It should be mentioned that the action of strychnia, when administered hypodermically, is far more powerful than when given by the mouth. In the treatment of strychnia-poisoning, emetics should be given at once, and the stomach-pump used if the lockjaw permits of it. Lockjaw can sometimes be overcome by chloroform, the administration of which is often attended in other respects with good results. The thirst can be relieved by strong tea better than anything else. Calabar bean, on account of being a spinal depressant, should be tried; and bromide of potassium in large doses, morphia, atropia, chloral hydrate, nitrite of amyl, may also prove efficacious as antidotes.

On post-mortem examination the brain and spinal cord may be found very much congested, with effusion of blood. Rigor mortis may be prolonged for several weeks after death. In extracting strychnia from the stomach the organic mixture should be first acidified with acetic acid, and sufficiently diluted to make filtering easy. The filtrate, having been evaporated to the consistency of a syrup, should be then heated with eight or ten times its bulk of alcohol, and again filtered, the liquid being distilled off. The filtrate should then be saturated with liquor potassæ and shaken up with its own bulk of ether. The acetate of strychnia, previously formed, being now decomposed by the potassa, the strychnia is precipitated and is taken up by the ether (Fig. 58). Any coloring-matter present may be removed by sulphuric acid. In order to insure the perfect purity of the strychnia, the above process should be repeated two or three times. Strychnia may be recognized

* Taylor: *op. cit.*, p. 224.

by its bitter taste, by the tetanic convulsions that it produces when injected subcutaneously into a frog, and by the play of colors it exhibits in the presence of nascent oxygen. It is probably the bitterest substance known. Indeed, it has been stated that one part of strychnia in seventy thousand parts of water gives a bitter taste.* In the absence, therefore, of such substances as morphia, quinia, aloes, colocynth, quassia, characterized also by having a bitter taste, a substance possessing this quality and alleged

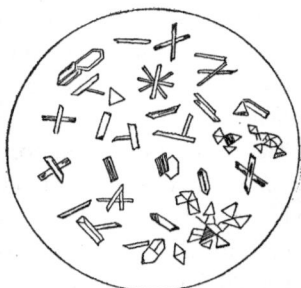

Fig. 58.—Various forms of crystals of strychnia from an ethereal solution.

to have caused death should certainly be tested still further for strychnia. The delicacy of the physiologic test—that is, of causing convulsions in a frog by the subcutaneous injection of strychnia—may be appreciated from the fact that convulsions follow the injection of only $\frac{1}{18000}$ part of a grain.†

The color test is performed by adding a drop of pure sulphuric acid to a small piece of strychnia on a white porcelain surface, the strychnia, if perfectly pure, being dissolved by the acid without coloration. If a little bichromate of potassium or binoxide of manganese be now stirred into the mixture, a play of colors will be presented, succeeding each other in the following order: blue, violet, purple, pink, and finally red. It should be observed that the value of the color test depends not so much upon any par-

* Guy and Ferrier: *op. cit.,* p. 562.
† Woodman and Tidy: *op. cit.,* p. 334.

ticular color being developed, or upon there being a play of colors, as upon the constant order in which the different colors manifest themselves. The color test is even more delicate than the physiologic one, the $\frac{1}{100000000000}$ of a grain of strychnia having been detected in this way.   It should be mentioned, however, that it has been objected that there are certain substances, like morphia, which interfere with the color test, and that there are other substances which exhibit very much the same play of colors on the addition of sulphuric acid.   In reply, it may be said that those substances which interfere with the color test can be gotten rid of by using chloroform instead of ether in extracting the alkaloid from the stomach, and that the change of color manifested by strychnia differs so much from that exhibited by other bodies on the addition of sulphuric acid that no real difficulty should be experienced in distinguishing them.

It may be mentioned that, in certain cases of poisoning by strychnia and other vegetable alkaloids, however thoroughly the analysis may be performed, the poison itself cannot be found.   As there is evidence that strychnia is decomposed in the system, its absence in those cases where there is every reason to believe it was administered can only be accounted for on the supposition that it was either eliminated in the excretion or, as in the case of opium, rejected by the stomach.

Brucia (Fig. 59), the remaining alkaloid of nux vomica, is usually found associated with strychnia.   As the symptoms of brucia are the same as those of strychnia, only less intense, and as the mode of extraction from the stomach is the same in the case of both alkaloids, we need not dwell upon its special properties.   It may be mentioned, however, that it turns to a blood-red color in the presence of nitric acid, the alkaloid being speedily dissolved.

Cerebro-spinal Neurotic Poisons :—*Deliriants.*—*Poisoning by Belladonna.*—Bella-donna may be considered as the type of a group of poisons the characteristic effects of which are frequently flushed face, redness of the skin, heat and dryness of the throat, dilatation of the pupil, illusion of the senses, and active delirium. Indeed, the latter symptom is so characteristic of these poisons that the entire group is often designated on that account as "deliriants." The group includes stramonium, hyoscyamus, different species of solanum as well as belladonna, all representatives of the natural order of Solanaceæ, and known therapeutically as *mydriatics*. The symptoms of poisoning by belladonna, the *Atropa belladonna* (Fig. 60) or deadly nightshade, appearing usually within two hours of taking the substance, are giddiness, drowsiness, intense thirst, dryness of the mouth and throat, difficulty in swallowing, the saliva being suppressed. Vomiting and purging are rare. The action of the heart is increased, pulse rapid and strong. The face is flushed, the eyes sparkle, with pupils invariably dilated. The power of speech is lost, though there is a constant movement of the lips and tongue, as if the patient were

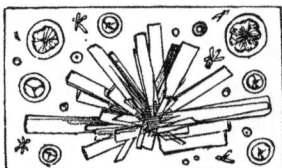

Fig. 59.—Crystals of brucia.

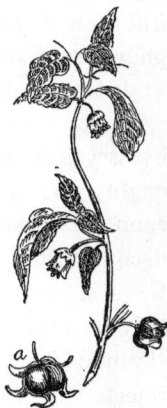

Fig. 60. — Atropa belladonna: *a*, The berry.

trying to articulate. Vision is affected, if not lost, through the loss of the power of accommodation. There is frequently a desire to micturate, with inability to do so. The patient is affected with all kinds of illusions and hallucinations, and finally with delirium, which in some cases may be of a pleasing character, in others so furious as to resemble mania. Death, when it occurs, takes place usually within twenty-four hours. A few berries of belladonna or a drachm of the extract have proved fatal.* The symptoms of poisoning by atropia, the active alkaloid of belladonna, are the same as those of the plant itself, but manifesting themselves more quickly and acting more powerfully. One and a half grains of atropia have proved fatal.†

In treating cases of poisoning by belladonna or atropia the stomach should be evacuated by an emetic or by means of the stomach-pump. Morphia should be administered hypodermically. As soon as the patient shows signs of getting better, castor oil may be given and strong coffee. The post-mortem appearances presented in cases of poisoning by atropia or belladonna are neither constant nor well marked. The pupils are dilated. The brain may be congested and the stomach inflamed. In cases of poisoning from belladonna, the remains of the leaves and berries should be carefully searched for in the stomach and intestines. Atropia can be extracted from the stomach by acidifying the contents of the latter with acetic acid and warm alcohol, and filtering. The filtrate should then be treated with subacetate of lead and sulphuretted hydrogen, by which the sulphide of lead is precipitated. The clear

* Woodman and Tidy: *op. cit.*, p. 410.
† Wharton and Stillé: *op. cit.*, p. 423.

filtrate evaporated to dryness and acidified, and saturated with potassa, can be then treated with alcohol, and the extract tested. A solution of hydrobromic acid saturated with free bromine gives a yellow precipitate which soon becomes crystalline, and is insoluble in mineral acids, acetic acid, or caustic alkalies. Atropia can also be tested by applying a portion of the extract to the eye of a man or of a rabbit, the smallest quantity producing dilatation of the pupil. As the symptoms, treatment, etc., of poisoning by stramonium or thornapple, Jamestown weed, hyoscyamus or henbane, Solanum dulcamara or bittersweet, woody nightshade, are essentially the same as those of belladonna, it will be unnecessary to dwell especially upon them.

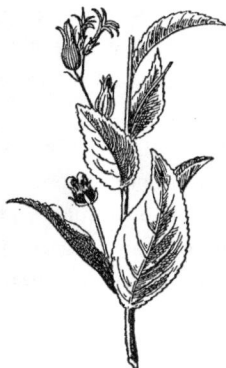

Fig. 61.—Lobelia inflata.

Depressants.—*Poisoning by Tobacco.*—Among the cerebro-spinal neurotic poisons are tobacco, lobelia (Fig. 61), conia, aconite, Calabar bean, often considered together on account of the property they possess in common of depressing the muscular system, although they may differ from one another in some respects. Tobacco, or the dried leaves of *Nicotiana tabacum*, owes its active and poisonous properties to a volatile liquid alkaloid, nicotina,* one of the most rapidly fatal poisons known, existing in Havana tobacco to an extent of only 2 per cent., but in Kentucky and Virginia tobaccos to as much as 7 per cent. The symptoms of poisoning by

* Tardieu: *op. cit.*, p. 778.

tobacco are giddiness, much depression and faintness, trembling of the limbs, clammy sweats, frequent vomiting, violent abdominal pains, with occasional purging. The pulse becomes first weak and then almost imperceptible; breathing becomes difficult; vision is affected; death taking place with convulsions and more or less paralysis. In treating cases of poisoning by tobacco, the stomach should be evacuated as soon as possible, either by emetics or the stomach-pump. Pain may be relieved by opium and the strength should be supported by stimulants. The external application of tobacco leaves and of a decoction of tobacco to the skin, as well as half a drachm given by enema, has proved fatal. Death has resulted from tobacco within fifteen minutes and from nicotina in three minutes.

On post-mortem examination the stomach, liver, lungs, and brain may be found congested, but not invariably. The remains of tobacco should be looked for with a lens, and the pieces examined under the microscope, the latter presenting a peculiar appearance on account of the hairs found upon them. In extracting tobacco from the stomach, essentially the same process may be used as that described in obtaining belladonna. A convenient test for nicotina is corrosive sublimate, which yields a white crystalline precipitate, soon changing to yellow, and soluble in acetic and hydrochloric acids. As the symptoms and post-mortem appearances caused by Indian tobacco, *Lobelia inflata*, or its active alkaloid, lobelina, are very much the same as those due to the taking of ordinary tobacco, it will be unnecessary to describe them. It may be mentioned, however, that one drachm of the powdered leaves has proved fatal in about thirty-six hours. On post-mortem examination the brain was found congested and the mucous membrane of the stomach inflamed.

Poisoning by conia, the active alkaloid of the spotted hemlock (*Conium maculatum*, Fig. 62), is generally the result of accident, the fresh leaves being sometimes used in cooking in mistake for parsley, which it slightly resembles. The symptoms are dryness and constriction of the throat, muscular prostration, pupils often dilated and vision affected; paralysis, and frequently convulsions, delirium,

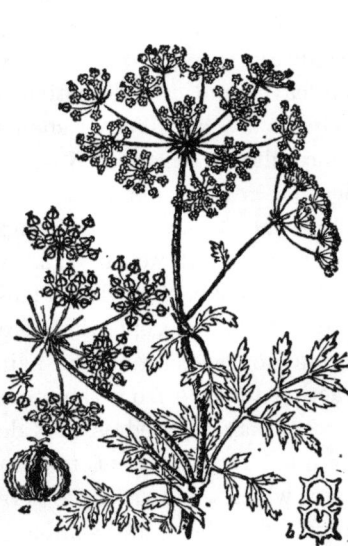

Fig. 62.—Conium maculatum : *a*, The fruit ; *b*, transverse section of the fruit.

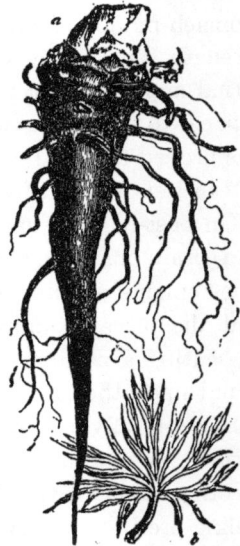

Fig. 63.—Aconitum napellus (aconite): *a*, The root ; *b*, the leaf.

and coma. The post-mortem appearances presented are those of asphyxia, congestion of the brain, and inflammation of the mucous membrane of the stomach. Treatment should consist in the administration of emetics, diffusible stimulants, and in practising artificial respiration.

Poisoning by Aconite.—The symptoms of poisoning by

aconite, obtained from monk's-hood or wolf's-bane (*Aconitum napellus*, Fig. 63), are dryness of the throat, with tingling and numbness of the lips and tongue, followed by nausea and vomiting and abdominal pain. There are ringing in the ears and diminishing, if not loss of, vision. The power of speech is lost. Breathing becomes slow and laborious. Cold, clammy sweats are common, accompanied with great prostration. The numbness of the limbs increases until finally both extremities are paralyzed. Death occurs either from shock, asphyxia, or syncope. Aconitia, the active alkaloid of aconite, is probably the most powerful poison known. In treating cases of poisoning by aconite or its active principle, an emetic of sulphate of zinc should be administered at once, or the stomach-pump used. Mustard plasters may be applied to the pit of the stomach; and ammonia, brandy, strong tea, or coffee should be given. Digitalis should be tried as an antidote. Twenty-five minims of Fleming's tincture and one-twentieth of a grain of aconite have proved fatal.* Death generally takes place within three or four hours; though it has occurred within twenty minutes, it has been delayed nearly twenty hours.

On post-mortem examination there is usually found general venous congestion, especially of the brain, liver, and lungs, as well as inflammation of the mucous membrane of the alimentary canal. The different parts of the plant should be carefully looked for. The process of extraction from the stomach is essentially the same as that described for obtaining belladonna. The characteristic symptoms produced when given to small animals, such as weakness, staggering, difficult breathing, convulsive twitch-

* Taylor: *op. cit.*, p. 226; Guy and Ferrier: *op. cit.*, p. 621.

ings, loss of sensibility, etc., constitute the most important tests for aconitia. Iodide of potassium may also be used as a test, giving with the alkaloid a reddish-brown amorphous precipitate.

The only case, so far as is known to the author, in which aconitia has been used with homicidal intent was that of the physician Lamson, who was tried, convicted, and executed in England, in 1882, for murdering his brother-in-law by means of this poison.

Calabar bean, the seed of *Physostigma venenosum*, owes its poisonous properties to an alkaloid, physostigma, or eserin. The symptoms of poisoning are giddiness, followed by paralysis of the voluntary muscles, convulsive muscular twitchings, and invariably contraction of the pupil. Owing to the latter property, atropia should be administered as an antidote. Six of the beans proved fatal in the case of a boy who had eaten them.*

Asthenics.—These poisons include not only the deliriant and depressant kinds of poisons, but also such as usually destroy life by causing heart failure, and hence often called "asthenics." The most important of this kind of poisons are hydrocyanic acid, digitalis, and cocculus indicus.

Poisoning by Hydrocyanic Acid.—Hydrocyanic or prussic acid is one of the most powerful and rapidly fatal poisons known, its effects being manifested with lightning-like rapidity. It is developed, rather than pre-existing, in the kernels of the peach, apricot, plum, cherry, and in the leaves and flowers of the peach and cherry-laurel through the action of water upon amygdalin and emulsin, two principles present in the plants. Pure prussic acid, being

* Woodman and Tidy: *op. cit.*, p. 320.

rarely found anywhere except in the laboratory of the chemist, has but little or no interest medico-legally. The medicinal acid, or the solution of the pure anhydrous acid in water, demands attention, however, on account of death being so frequently caused by it.

The symptoms produced by prussic-acid poisoning are giddiness, with immediate loss of muscular power, the person staggering and falling to the ground. The breathing becomes quick and gasping, the pulse imperceptible. The eyes protrude and are glassy, the pupils being dilated and insensible to light. The extremities are cold. The face becomes livid or pale. The jaws are spasmodically closed. There may be bloody frothing at the mouth, and the odor of the poison may be noticed on the breath. Death may take place preceded by coma, stertorous breathing, or by convulsions. Unfortunately, the poisonous effects of prussic acid manifest themselves so quickly that the opportunity is but rarely afforded for treatment. The latter, when practicable, consists in applying cold affusions, practising artificial respiration, placing ammonia to the nostrils. A mixture of a ferrous and ferric sulphate of iron with caustic alkali should be administered with the hope of forming the inert ferrocyanide of potassium. Emetics and the stomach-pump should also be used. On post-mortem examination the lungs, liver, spleen, and kidneys will be found gorged with blood. The brain may be found congested, and there may be effusion of serum into the ventricles. The stomach and intestines may also be found congested. The most important, constant, and characteristic sign noticed, however, is the distinct odor of prussic acid exhaled when the body is opened and often even before it is opened. Fifty minims of the official acid, equivalent to about nine-tenths of a grain of the anhydrous acid, have proved fatal.* Death may occur either instantaneously or within ten or fifteen minutes after swallowing the poison, being rarely protracted half an hour.

The general method adopted in extracting prussic acid from the stomach is to distil the contents of the latter at a gentle heat, the vapor being collected in a receiver kept cool by being placed in cold water, or to acidify the contents of the stomach if alkaline, and place the mixture in a vessel standing in a basin containing water at 60° F., and then testing the rising vapor. The presence of prussic acid can be recognized by the white cyanide of silver formed through application of nitrate of silver, by the white sulphocyanide of ammonium formed with sulphide of ammonium, the latter turning red on the addition of perchloride of iron, the formation of Prussian blue by adding liquor potassæ, a proto- and per-salt of iron, and sulphuric acid. As the symptoms, etc., of poisoning by the cyanides, oil of bitter almonds, cherry-laurel water, the kernels of the peach, apricot, and cherry, essence of mirbane, are essentially the same as those produced by prussic acid proper, only less intense, they need not be especially considered.

Poisoning by Digitalis.—The symptoms of poisoning by foxglove (*Digitalis purpurea*, Fig. 64), or its active alkaloid, digitalin, are headache, giddiness, nausea, vomiting, purging, abdominal pain, dimness of vision with dilated pupils, slow, irregular pulse. In treating cases of poisoning by digitalis, emetics should be given, and infusions containing tannin, such as tea, coffee, oak bark, etc., as stimulants. On post-mortem examination the brain may

* Woodman and Tidy: *op. cit.*, p. 457.

be found congested, and the mucous membrane of the stomach inflamed. Digitalis may be extracted from the stomach by the process used in obtaining belladonna. The most reliable test for digitalin is the effect it produces upon the action of the frog's heart, causing stoppage and irregularity in the beats.

Poisoning by Cocculus Indicus. —The symptoms of poisoning by *cocculus indicus,* or the berry of *Anamirta cocculus,* a genus of the Menispermaceæ, or the moonseed order, are gastro-intestinal irritation, accompanied with lethargic stupor and powerlessness. The poisonous properties are due to an alkaloid, picrotoxin. Of six persons poisoned accidentally on one occasion by a decoction of cocculus indicus, two died within half an hour, the remaining four recovering after several hours. The prominent symptoms in these cases were giddiness, faintness, nausea, dimness of vision, intense thirst, and abdominal pain.*

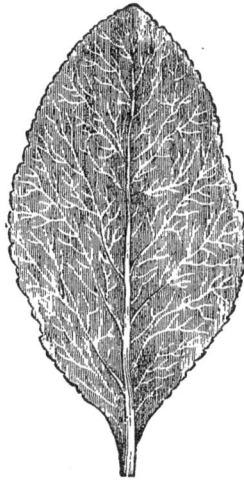

Fig. 64.—Digitalis purpurea leaf.

In conclusion, it may be mentioned that the laburnum (*Cytisus laburnum*), the yew (*Taxus baccata*), the privet (*Legistrum vulgare*), the Guelder rose (*Viburnum opulus*), and the holly (*Ilex aquifolium*) possess acrid, irritant, narcotic properties even when eaten in small quantities.

* Wharton and Stillé: *op. cit.,* vol. ii, p. 499.

INDEX.